Growing up with HIV in Zimbabwe

Cover photograph: Linette Frewin
First published by Africaid in their exhibition 'The Audacity of Hope',
World AIDS day, 2010 and reproduced here with their kind permission.
We would also like to thank Tsvangirai Mukwazhi for his photograph on page 122,
Irene Staunton for the photograph on page 170 and Linette Frewin for all
other photographs, and for her generous support of this project.
© Photograph on p. 122 Tsvangirai Mukwazhi
©Photograph on p. 170 Irene Staunton
© Photographs on pp. 1, 17, 52, 92, 149 Linette Frewin

Growing up with HIV in Zimbabwe

One day this will all be over

Ross Parsons

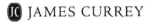

James Currey
is an imprint of Boydell & Brewer Ltd
PO Box 9, Woodbridge, Suffolk IP12 3DF, GB
www.jamescurrey.com
and of
Boydell & Brewer Inc.
668 Mt Hope Avenue, Rochester, NY 14620-2731, US
www.boydellandbrewer.com

Weaver Press
PO Box A1922
Avondale
Harare
Zimbabwe
www.weaverpress.co.zw

Published in paperback in Zimbabwe and Southern Africa by Weaver Press under
the title *One Day this will all be Over: Growing up with HIV in urban Eastern Zimbabwe*
and published in cloth in the rest of the world by James Currey under the title
Growing up with HIV in Zimbabwe: One Day this will all be Over

1 2 3 4 5 15 14 13 12

British Library Cataloguing in Publication Data
A catalogue record for this book is available from the British Library

ISBN 978-1-84701-048-3 (James Currey Cloth)

Papers used by Boydell & Brewer are natural, recyclable products
made from wood grown in sustainable forests

Typeset in Linotype Didot 10.5/15pt by forzalibro designs, Harare
Printed and bound in Great Britain by CPI Group (UK) Ltd, Croydon, CR0 4YY

Contents

Preface and acknowledgements

'For how can I go so far as to try to use language
to get between pain and its expression?'

Ludwig Wittgenstein
Philosophical Investigations (1945: 245)

The following is a work haunted by suffering and grief. I offer it as an inadequate memorial to the children I have known who have now died. I am greatly indebted to all the children and their families whom I have come to know, indeed to acknowledge as my own, in the course of the work. I have gone to great lengths to obscure their identities in what follows but I hope not to have obscured their great generosity of spirit, of resilience and of their consummate good humour.

In Zimbabwe, Dr Geoff Foster, Dr Mark Patterson and the paediatric staff at Mutare Provincial Hospital were more than hospitable and I have the greatest respect for their commitment, dedication and hard work. Dr Thokozile Chitepo, Dr Isaac Machakanja, Dr Abigail Kangwende and Mrs Maryjoice Kapesa, in the Faculty of Humanities and Social Sciences at Africa University, provided a congenial intellectual home amidst the general degradation of Zimbabwean academia. Michael Bourdillon, Professor Emeritus of Anthropology at the University of Zimbabwe, is always a kind and generous colleague who shares with me his encyclopedic knowledge of local ethnographic literature and reads earlier drafts of work. Nancy Chulu maintained the children's group with great equanimity and compassion during my absences. Hellen Magadaire was an invaluable research assistant and translator at various points. Ashleigh Mortelman very generously gave the final manuscript a thorough proofreading, which greatly helped me in the final stages of preparing the manuscript. She also generously helped me in my understanding of, and admiration for, Pentecostal Christianity.

In the USA, the work was funded, fostered and supported by the Department of Anthropology at The Johns Hopkins University where faculty and fellow students helped me greatly in clarifying, deepening and widening my thinking. In particular, I am deeply grateful to Pamela Reynolds, Jane Guyer and Aaron Goodfellow who were diligent, generous and provocative interlocutors. Sylvain Perdigon, Sidharthan Maunaguru, Valeria Procupez and Vaibhav Saria are all both great friends and immensely helpful readers. Paola Maratti and Ruth Leys in the Department of Humanities, and Sara Berry and Pier Larson in the Department of History all read drafts, commenting and teaching with the greatest generosity. In particular earlier drafts of a number of chapters were greatly improved by their reception in the university's Africa Seminar and Anthropology Colloquia. Any errors are entirely my own.

Amanda Hammar, in the Centre for African Studies at the University of Copenhagen, whose seminal work in Zimbabwean studies has been one of my inspirations, has long been one of my most valued friends and colleagues. Fiona Ross, in the Department of Social Anthropology at the University of Cape Town, has provoked and supported my work at a number of crucial junctures. Jane Reece, at the University of Bristol and a fellow traveller, has been a friend, editor and encourager.

Irene Staunton and Murray McCartney at Weaver Press in Harare have been strong supporters of the publication of the manuscript and facilitated its acceptance by Douglas Johnson at James Currey/

Boydell and Brewer. Helpful readers' reports, which greatly improved the manuscript, were provided by Sara Berry and Amanda Hammar. I have also been very privileged to work with the Zimbabwean photographer, Linette Frewin, an old friend, whose photographs of HIV-positive Zimbabwean children add immeasurably to the final book.

Yogesh Nathoo, *meri jaan*, has endured, more than anyone else, my long preoccupation with the work. None of it would have been possible without his love, generosity and support.

1

Introduction
Growing up with HIV in urban, eastern Zimbabwe

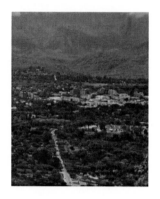

Why, and how, do HIV-positive children sometimes survive in the midst of the multiple deprivations and extreme social suffering associated with living in contemporary Zimbabwe? What does such survival look like? Zimbabwe stands at the epicentre of a regional, indeed global, HIV pandemic. Infection rates are variously estimated at over 14% and the weekly mortality rate is said to approach 4,000 (more on the problems of statistics later). Child survival from HIV is rare. Most HIV-positive children will die before the age of five, and this remains the case even after the advent of antiretroviral drugs. To explore the questions in an ethnographic mode I established regular contact with a group of children in the eastern Zimbabwean border town of Mutare, all of whom were HIV-positive. Details of the children, their circumstances and the ways through which I came to know them are described in full in the following chapter. In the constant presence of ambivalence towards the multiple adversities of life, these children embody a fierce attachment to a daily life that is staked as free from the dilemmas inherited at birth and confronted each day. And yet a strong attachment may have its limits.

The indicators of the contemporary Zimbabwean crisis are widely known: inter alia, unemployment estimated around 90%, hyperinflation approaching 14,000% (prior to dollarization in early 2009), life expectancy declined to the mid-30s (from the mid-70s two decades ago), widespread state-sponsored violence and the denial of fundamental democratic rights, hunger and food insecurity, and decaying state institutions (Raftopoulos and Mlambo 2009, Hammar, Raftopoulos and Jensen 2003, Raftopoulos and Savage 2004, Harold-Barry 2004, Alexander 2006, Hammar, McGregor and Landau 2010, Jones 2010, Musoni 2010, Worby 2010).[1]

The children I worked with lived under the shadow of untimely death, unexpectedly and indeterminately deferred. Physically small for their ages, they often bore the outward signs of affliction and illness, and constantly stood exposed to the unstable, potentially devastating possibilities of social stigma and rejection. Their survival, however, indicates that for some, care has been found, and

---

[1] The indicators I give here were correct in 2008/9, when this section was written. The Zimbabwean situation is highly fluid, and there have been numerous changes. Dollarization has brought relative price stability, and schools and health institutions have been partially resuscitated under the Government of National Unity (GNU). There have been two outbreaks of cholera and one of measles with large and entirely preventable fatalities. Political violence has begun to rise again in anticipation of an imminent referendum on a new Constitution and a national election. There are three main sources for information and analysis about Zimbabwe. Firstly, the news media based both in and outside the country. Personally I find the weekly *Zimbabwe Independent*, the *Mail and Guardian* (a South African weekly) and *The Guardian* (a London daily) to be the most reliable and consistent in their coverage. Secondly the invaluable work of documentation carried out primarily by churches and non-governmental organizations. The many and detailed reports of the Solidarity Peace Trust are the richest in detail and narrative depth (www.solidaritypeacetrust.org). Thirdly there is a burgeoning academic literature, emanating from both in and outside the country. For the most recent and critical contributions see Hammar et al. (2010), especially articles by Jones, Musoni 2010 and Worby 2010. See also Orner and Holmes (2010), a remarkable and richly nuanced collection of personal narratives across a wide range of Zimbabwean society.

is perhaps more available than we might have thought. Recently initiated into a (chaotic) national rollout of antiretroviral treatment programmes, these children are strikingly ambivalent about such treatments, favouring the possibilities of supernatural healing, often through charismatic Pentecostal churches (Maxwell 2006, Robbins 2004).

The study observed, amongst much else, grief, ambivalence, shame, resistance, and persistence in the face of death. The emotions had social expressions and intimate textures and were instantiated in the daily lives of children. The children lived with self-imposed secrecy and selective confession, strategic engagements with kin and their peers, and through their performances, effacements and self-representations in public spaces and activities. My previous training as a psychotherapist, and established relationships of trust, allowed me to approach the difficult task of working with chronically ill children with an ethical sensitivity, a careful artisanship, and a complementary theoretical and methodological base, that brought to bear the two disciplines of anthropology and psychology on the subject at hand.[2]

My psychotherapeutic work formed a foundation, and a parallel endeavour, that allowed me to move outwards from a therapeutic setting to develop an ethnographic portrait of children growing up in a small African urban centre under conditions of extreme adver-

[2]   The relationship between the two disciplines has a long history. Malinowski (for example, 1966) engaged actively with Freudian concepts as did many of his students. Margaret Mead (1928) used Freud too in her critique of American child upbringing via the adolescents of Western Samoa. Following her was the substantial work of the American school of 'personality and culture' in anthropology. More recently there has been a return to the post-Freudian and Lacanian literatures as a means of developing anthropological theory. For example see Henrietta Moore (2007) and Suzette Heald and Ariane Deluz (1994). The relationship is not restricted to psychoanalysis. Cognitive psychology has had a close relationship with linguistic anthropology and queer theory, especially the work of Sedgwick (2003, for example) has reanimated interest in Sylvan Tompkins's affect theory.

sity. The children's lives are lived within the imbrications of poverty, multiple bereavements, displacements, and disruptions in schooling, and the care associated with normative notions of kinship having been complicated by living with a chronic, life-threatening illness. Resources, whether practical or emotional, were few given the ongoing depletion and decline of the Zimbabwean state. I deliberately chose a small urban centre as the site of the study, because we know that the population of sub-Saharan Africa is both young and rapidly urbanizing.[3] The ethnographic material permits me to look back, from the standpoint of the children and their carers, at the institutions in which their lives are suspended and through which they are mediated: government clinics and schools (now sorely depleted, but still offering some continuity of care, at least in Mutare), and the moralizing forces and funding agencies of international NGOs and their local partners. What do global HIV prevention and treatment organizations, and the care they provide, look like through the eyes of a child?

HIV research and intervention organizations, and the care they provide, partially escaped the more draconian forms of state surveillance and control imposed on international donor funding agencies within contemporary Zimbabwean autarky, so their operations are ubiquitous in the lives of the HIV-positive children and their families. International and local NGOs (many of which are faith-based) working on the HIV pandemic continue to be relatively well funded and highly active in Manicaland, in eastern Zimbabwe, and across the country. The category of the orphan and the vulnerable child has assumed the status of a universal value, a marker of international

---

[3] I would argue that African studies has been historically marked, indeed stunted, by a serious excess of questionable generalizations. Here is the first of my own (however, see annual reports of the World Bank on Africa: www.worldbank.org/annualreports for some justification). If there is such a thing as a general social trend, this may be an important one. The exceptions to trends though are both most often overlooked and yet most revealing.

acknowledgement of extreme need, and may act to allow access to donor funding and support for families and communities (and the state itself), or occlude other life-sustaining forms of care.[4] A psychotherapeutically informed ethnography contextualizes and personalizes the figure of the orphan (vulnerable, isolated, dangerously unsocialized) as a globally iconic figure of crisis in contemporary Africa.[5]

Bodies of literature

The growing body of scholarship on the anthropology of childhood (Das and Reynolds 2003, Reynolds 1995/2000, Scheper-Hughes 1992, for example) has revealed aporia in the ethnographic record surrounding the lives and social worlds of children. In these works children emerge as more than passive innocents, and as actors and strategists in domestic relations, as labourers and as contributors to households. The literature is not monolithic; for example, Scheper-Hughes and Sargent (1998) emphasize with urgency a growing debate around universal rights for children, while others (Reynolds 1995; Das and Reynolds 2003; Niewenhuys 1996), with close attention to local social worlds, find such universality problematic and

---

[4] See Foster et al. (2005) *A generation at risk: The global impact of HIV/AIDS on orphans and vulnerable children* for an influential edited volume on 'orphans and vulnerable children in Africa'.

[5] See Castaneda (2000) for an extraordinary account of the way in which children and children's bodies have been used as 'figures' (powerful though partially hidden) in a variety of literatures. Castaneda argues forcibly that the child is a flexible figure, always becoming, and always available as the screen on which society may project a range of discourses, anxieties and projects. Here the actual living child is not at stake, rather, what is at stake is the figure of the child as a highly malleable container for a range of social and intellectual projects of becoming. For the most influential account of 'the crisis' in Africa see Mbembe (2001, 2002) and Mbembe and Roitman (1995). The idea of 'the crisis' as a social and temporal zone can, I think, be attributed to Giorgio Agamben (1998, 1999).

stress the interwoven realities of children's work and the choices they face as contributors to households. Within Africa, the study of childhoods has been given new urgency by the appearance of children as soldiers, migrants and other liminal figures (Honwana and De Boeck 2005, Honwana 2006). The renewed sense of the importance surrounding children's lives recalls Malinowski's (1966) proposition that the family, however variously constituted, pivots on the lynchpin of the child.

The ethnographic literature on children in Africa can be usefully juxtaposed against a background of the phenomenology of experience as mediated through emotions (Desjarlais 1993/2003, Lutz 1988, Lutz and White 1986, Sedgwick 2003) and the body (Csordas 1994, Desjarlais 1993/2003). The emotions that constitute the everyday (Das 1990/1996) are heightened when considered against the grain of social suffering, violence and bare life; tropes commonly deployed to understand the lives of children in zones pictured as socially abandoned (Biehl 2005, Mbembe 2001, Agamben 1998/1999).

The bridge between the two bodies of literature might be found in the anthropology of illness (Kleinman 1988, Farmer 2003) especially that dealing with chronic illness and the exacerbation of suffering brought about through structural violence (Farmer 2003). Local African healing traditions provide a persistent template of social response to illness experiences within local contexts (Feierman and Janzen 1992). The notion of 'bare life' is problematized here: the 'bare' is seen to abound with unexpected contingencies.[6] The con-

[6] Once again, see the influential work of Agamben (1998, 1999) in relation to the notion of 'bare life', which is partially based on a very selective reading of Levi (for example, 1988) and his description of the 'grey zone' in the Nazi death camps. The idea has been used by Biehl (2005) in relation to poverty and HIV in Brazil, and by Mbembe (2001) in relation to decay and conflict in African societies. I suggest that my ethnography undermines the idea of 'the bare': social life even under severe poverty and widespread social violence appears to have stronger resources and greater resilience. (See Chapter 6).

cept of psychological trauma is therefore especially problematized (Leys 2000), as is normative western developmental psychology which fails to account for the survival, development and indeed the becoming adult of children who mature within contexts of severe adversity (Burman 2008). Anthropology is well placed, perhaps even impelled, to make important contributions to understanding such wide variations of experience as is evidenced by the discipline's history (see, for example, Mead 1928).

In African scholarly literatures the figure of the child has been both amplified and problematized by work that focuses on the different forms social estrangement may take locally. For example, de Boeck (1998) has traced the lives of Congolese children through a wide range of marginal and non-childlike activities as, for example, illegal miners, child soldiers, exiles from family structures and self-confessed devotees of the occult. Indeed the ambiguous engagement of children with the occult resonates elsewhere in the regional literature (Geschiere and Roitman 1997, Ashforth 2005). In contrast, writing from within the HIV pandemic in South Africa, Henderson (2004) is developing work that depicts children as survivors through the tenacious persistence of normality. My project also focuses on the mundane and quotidian lives of children, examining their surprising persistence, and their careful avoidance of liminal markings.

The child orphan operates as a figure (Castaneda 2002) in the literature which gestures towards the extreme vulnerability and/or danger of the liminal child (Turner 1967/1981, Meintjies and Giese 2006, Reynolds 2000). Living in states of chronic and life-threatening illness heightens their liminality (Bluebond-Langner 1978, Phillips 1993/2000, Scheper-Hughes 1992), although Myra Bluebond-Langner speaks more directly to child deaths closely mediated by institutions (such as hospitals), which is less the case in Zimbabwe. However, the institutions themselves deserve considerable scrutiny as sites of the moral, and as actors in 'gift' economies (Bornstein 2006, Russ 2005, Mauss 1967).

An extensive psychoanalytic literature applies to the project of understanding emotion, and its imbrications in close relationships and attachments. The literature includes Freud (2005) on ambivalence, and repetition, mourning and melancholia; Ferenczi (1955) on the 'unwanted child' and Winnicott (1958) on 'the unheld'. There is a long history of engagement between anthropology and psychoanalysis (for example, Rivers 1926, Sapir 1949, Kardiner and Linton 1939, Devisch and Brodeur 1999, Heald and Deluz 1994, and Bateson 1958/1972). This is directly relevant to an understanding of the interface between the social and the psychological (Menzies-Lyth 1988/1989), which is central to my proposition that anthropology and psychotherapy have capacities (as yet relatively undeveloped) to explicate the lives of children, and the stakes entailed in their transfiguration into adults, under conditions of extreme adversity.

Further there is, within anthropology and area studies, a regional southern and central African literature of some provenance and theoretical weight which presents the family in specific ways (Gluckman 1955, Turner 1967/1981, Richards 1939, Gelfand 1979, Bourdillon 1991, Ferguson 1999, Reynolds 1995/2000, Ross 2003) and is invested in the modes of analysis interpellated with the tropes of the post-colonial and the historical (Comaroff 1992, Mbembe 2001, Van Onselen 1996), but is nonetheless a participant in the aporia surrounding childhoods (with the exception of Reynolds 1995/2005). Newer work highlights the growing importance of an explosively growing Pentecostal Christianity (Maxwell 2006) with powerful promises of healing, echoing, yet superseding, older regional healing cults (Ranger 1999, Werbner 1977/1997, Feierman and Janzen 1992). The literature on religion and healing is highly relevant to daily life in Mutare which follows much of the rest of Africa in witnessing the power of syncretic healing practices and where the children I worked with participate in various types of ritual practices.

Anthropologists have begun to grapple with the challenge of producing an ethnography of decline (Ferguson 1999) in contexts where the possibilities of the post-colonial moment have been seriously eroded through a combination of poor local governance and international, globalizing late capitalism (Mbembe 2001, Ferguson 2006). Relatedly, it is important for anthropology to make careful commentary in response to the growing, hegemonic public health literature on the HIV pandemic in southern Africa: the figures of the orphan and the caregiver, the contexts of activism, and the 'intervention' of psychosocial support (Henderson 2004, Meintjies 2005, Foster et al. 2000).

The structure of the ethnography

My purpose in fieldwork was to obtain as full a picture as possible of the lives of children growing up with HIV in Mutare, a town in eastern Zimbabwe. The project included close observation of their lives within their families, and in relation to the clinics and churches they attend. Crucially, I tried to understand their relationships to death: the threat of their own deaths, the heavy weight of the bereavements they bore and the unrelenting grieving that life offered them.

In Chapter 2 I describe the site of the study, Mutare (an eastern border town). Intermingled with both physical and historical description, I demonstrate the constant presence of religious motifs that point to a sense of sorrow and loss, often rendered in the poetries of spiritual language. I also describe the children I came to know during the course of the study, and the methodologies (all within the registers of the ethnographic) through which I undertook my explorations. Central to the work were questions of ethics, heightened by being witness to everyday extremity in the context of a failing state. I explore ways in which such questions became central to my practice as a researcher.

In Chapter 3 I explore children's experiences of care within their families and wider kin structures. The exploration requires a close reading of the history of kinship theory within Zimbabwean anthropological writing which, in turn, needs to be contextualized within the colonial (and post-colonial) political contexts within which it was produced. Experiences of care are examined through ethnographic material that attends to quotidian terrains of domesticity, which include instantiations of marriage, familial loss, and the provision of food, amongst much else. The material reveals a constantly shifting tension between idealized notions of family, kin and care and everyday experiences of loss, shortcoming and privation.

Chapter 4 takes up the central issue of children's experiences of illnesses. These take on a variety of forms (almost always life-threatening) and leave a variety of bodily inscriptions. I claim that infection with HIV is lived as an intense secret despite its obvious physical manifestations and, yet, in a way that does not entirely occlude forms of sustaining sociality. Perhaps, I suggest, infection with HIV is experienced less as chronic illness than as vulnerability to multiple, random illnesses all of which impinge heavily and unpredictably on abilities to survive in a ruthless world in which sharp social reflexes and constant adaptation are essential. I offer a particular focus here on the role of the local paediatric clinic in offering partial medical care against a background of daunting resource constraints. I also suggest that western forms of medical care are encountered by children against a template of other ideas about illness and healing. Such ideas include those with roots in traditional forms of healing as well as, more importantly, those that arise within contexts of intense engagement with various forms of Christianity.

The roles of religious practices, especially in a plethora of Christian forms, as mediators of dire experience forms the substance of Chapter 5. Central to the chapter is ethnographic material that explores ideas about faith and healing in contexts of devout belief as manifested through practice. The resurgence of Christian churches in contemporary Zimbabwe can hardly be over-emphasized. Here I examine churches in Mutare and the variety of roles they play for the children. Faith-healing is particularly emphasized within churches in the charismatic/Pentecostal spectrum, but is also to be found in older independent Zionist formations. Ideas about healing, particularly those usually subsumed under the rubric of the 'traditional', are often manifested in common knowledge about local medicinal herbs and related pharmacopoeia. Healing is but one aspect, though, of religious fervour. Theodicy[7] is immersed and countered in a fervent, almost mystical, relationship to ideas about a suffering yet loving God.

Chapter 6 attempts a confrontation with experiences of death, dying and grief. The ethnographic material is deeply painful. I argue that spiritual belief about a loving God and a peaceful afterlife is reinforced by grief-stricken memories about lost loved ones to make death preferable to continued suffering. Idioms of despair and resignation haunt children as they actively resign from partial medical care, and retire to sites of social withdrawal in preparation for their deaths. Such idioms draw on both 'traditional' and Christian imagery in their evocative power. I suggest that it is possible that scripture and prayer provide children with words with which to bridge the unspeakable. Contemporary theories of grief, drawn from a western psychology, provide little help in an understanding of the experiences explored here.

In an epilogue, Chapter 7, I offer a partial conclusion to the ethnography. I return to an ethic of restraint (more follows on this) but offer the outlines of two sets of concluding ideas. The first addresses discourses of the body and of HIV, primarily in anthropology. The second suggests some avenues for thinking through the com-

---

[7] Theodicy refers to a central problem in theology, which is how to explain or understand the existence of suffering if there is a benevolent and all-powerful deity. It was most clearly articulated by Leibnitz (1710) but is a problem of considerable antiquity and, obviously, remains unresolved. In modern times, the idea was shown to be intricately imbricated in social life through the influential work of Max Weber (1905), who also extended the problem to polytheistic religions.

plicated, but potentially rich, interface between anthropology and psychoanalysis. Neither discipline, it seems to me, currently offers clear theoretical pathways for thinking through the experiences of sociality in contexts of mass death and severe adversity.

Ethnography, evidence and an ethic of restraint

I contend that, in the presence of wholesale death and suffering, it is incumbent on us to approach the material I offer here with an ethic of restraint. I had believed that the phrase was my own, borne from a long contemplation of the sheer, if banal, horror I had witnessed. Recently I discovered that the phrase must be attributed to the Dalai Lama (1999), although our uses of the term are different in intent and emphasis. I use the phrase to imply that scholars and activists might find a respectful yet fulsome witness. Analysis may be both unseemly and premature under the circumstances. Through the notion of restraint I specifically mean that we need to stop short of burdening lives and deaths with an immediate recourse to theoretical analysis and policy formulation. We need to be quiet and still, and to find (as I will suggest later) an appropriate pause prior to interpretation. I take the idea of 'an interpretive pause' from Marilyn Strathern (1996) and develop my use of it more fully in Chapter 6.

The ethic here is, perhaps, one common to all of the anthropology of social suffering. It is a dilemma heightened by the stringent demands of writing ethnography of which Clifford Geertz had the following to say:

> There are three characteristics of ethnographic description: it is interpretive; what it is interpretive of is the flow of social discourse; and the interpreting involved consists in trying to rescue the 'said' of such discourse from its perishing occasions and fix it in perusable terms ... there is, in addition, a fourth characteristic ... it is microscopic. (Geertz 1973: 20)

The 'perishing occasions' here are quite literal and certainly micro-scopic. A few child deaths amongst so many are tragic but might be questioned as empirical evidence, especially as I insist throughout on the local specificity of my knowledge. The empirical has many forms and is itself the subject of much debate and many interpretations. By referencing Clifford Geertz I align myself with one trajectory of in-terpretations. Geertz's 'thick description' (taken, with acknowledge-ment, from Gilbert Ryle, 1971) implies that ethnography is produced through placing the speech of informants within descriptions of an ever-widening and deepening social context. I have followed this model. A significant part of such descriptions is a reliance on previ-ous anthropological work. As we shall see, earlier anthropologists were not afraid of generalizations. In this study, I rely heavily on the works of J.F. Holleman, M.F.C. Bourdillon and others, because they initiated the study of what has come to be known as Shona culture. The generalizations seem excessive now but I cannot apologize for the anthropological canon. I can only hope to enrich it with specific-ity in a small way.

My ethnography relies heavily on the close knowledge and detailed description of a small group of children. Indeed the reader will find that some children are more closely rendered than others. In this I follow a long tradition both within anthropology (Crapanzano 1985, Biehl 2005, for example) and psychology (particularly in the Freud-ian traditions) of using the particular to suggest the more general. I would go further to suggest that it is the dilemma of all writing. As the novelist Marguerite Yourcenar (1984 [1929]) said through her protagonist, Alexis:

> A letter, even the longest, is obliged to simplify what should not have been simplified: one is always so much less clear the minute one tries to be complete. I should like to make here an effort not only of sin-cerity but also of precision: hence, these pages will contain many erasures; they do already. (Yourcenar 1984: 3)

Shock, witnessing and grief

The difficulties of writing the material are further confounded by the element of shock inherent in the work. Certainly the fieldwork caused me to be shocked and I think it will many readers. The 'shock' arises out of both the context and the process I describe here. By process I mean the forms the ethnography took, and therefore the paths by which it ended up in the form it has. For example, beginning the research, I had imagined that I would devote considerable attention to children's experiences within schools. The absolute collapse of the Zimbabwean educational system (towards the later 2000s) rendered this redundant during the time period of the study. By context I refer to the overarching contexts of children's lives. In particular, I refer to the ongoing collapse of the Zimbabwean state and the real effects of that collapse on the lives of poor, urban, HIV-positive children.

The shocking suffering faced by children I describe, therefore, gives rise in the researcher to a certain form of witnessing. By witnessing I mean processes of observing, recording and contextualizing that are central elements of ethnographic practice, but are also central to becoming enmeshed with local social realities. 'Enmeshed' might also suggest a certain 'being messed up by'. For me, the form of witnessing that results resonates with the witnessing described by Veena Das in 'Our work to cry, your work to listen' (1990) in which, in the wake of communal riots in India, she suggests new forms of witnessing that are constructed in part by the horror of experience and the distanced position of (professional) observers. For me, a certain important difference lies in my experience of both listening to and crying with the accounts of my informants.

Shock and witnessing, therefore, urge attention to forms of grief and mourning. The work I present here, as I shall point out in detail later, poses severe challenges to established models of grief and mourning within western psychology and within forms of anthropol-

14

ogy (even those that have, in recent years, urged a new concentration on 'social suffering'). Mass death and bereavement, especially when thoroughly grounded in a banal everyday, challenge established theoretical models. I have found myself groping towards the literatures of the Holocaust in search of appropriate parallels (although I do not think the Holocaust is one).

For me (as a result of a particular background in psychotherapy) the questions I pose above strongly suggest a re-examination of psychoanalysis, as a theoretical resource rather than as a technique of practice. Central to Freud's insights was the claim that misery in life is unavoidable. For him it was a matter of neurotic misery (which might be ameliorated) and common unhappiness (which was simply the lot of humankind). These were insights, however, developed in contexts of western European bourgeois urbanity. In this regard psychoanalysis too falls short of the enormity of suffering at stake here. However, what else might be at stake in a psychoanalytically inflected ethnography? I suggest we might consider the following: going along with the suffering (a certain form of companionship), insisting on spaces of observation, pausing before interpretations, and tolerating pain, uselessness and horror.

It is from such considerations that my suggestion of an ethic of restraint arises as a form of deliberate hesitation before the headlong rush to policy and practice. In this sense, I write in the pause that falls between observation and reaction. Whatever comes next (and every chapter I present here suggests avenues for further urgent examination), I think that much current writing in anthropology about living (and dying) with HIV requires detailed consideration in other contexts. As I shall suggest in my epilogue, influential writing in medical anthropology (such as that by João Biehl, 2005, 2007, and Arthur Kleinman, 1988, 2006) hinges on claims of redemption and recuperation being possible through the practice of western medicine unhindered by resource constraints. My work suggests otherwise. It would seem to me to be hubris to seek full social or individual recuperation in the face of chronic illness through western bio-medicine. Lives are constituted by much more than their engagement (or not) with either medical practice or humanitarian intervention.

2

In this vale of tears
An ethnography of suffering and sorrow

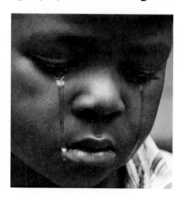

Introduction

In the course of my fieldwork I have attended too many funerals. In late 2008 I attended the funeral of a boy in one of Mutare's Catholic churches. The congregation sang, with piercing sweetness and haunting plaintiveness, the Salve Regina, a traditional hymn to Mary. In their version the recurring phrase was 'we are banished in this vale of tears'. The hymn's words are:

> Hail, holy Queen, mother of mercy!
> Our light, our sweetness and our hope!
> To you do we cry, poor banished children of Eve, to you do we send up our sighs, mourning and weeping in this vale of tears.
> Turn then, most gracious advocate, your eyes of mercy towards us; and after this our exile, show unto us the blessed fruit of your womb, Jesus.
> O clement, o loving, o sweet virgin Mary.[1]

---

[1]   An old Roman Catholic Marian prayer, attributed to a monk of the Middle Ages, Hermann of Reichenau, that remains in frequent and widespread use.

At that moment the landscape and the hymn and the terrible sense of loss all coalesced, for me, into a moment full of many sorrows and losses. I take this phrase, 'the vale of tears' as an appropriate entry into a description of the place and form of this study.

The site of the study: histories and landscapes

The study was undertaken in Mutare, a small, dusty, provincial town. At least 'town' is what both its inhabitants and the casual observer would refer to it as. Here I want to give a detailed description of the place, as the site of ethnographic enquiry, and to document the way in which the study was formulated and undertaken. Officially, since 1971, it has been a (self-proclaimed) city, provincial capital of Zimbabwe's easternmost province of Manicaland, and the site of the most important border crossing between Zimbabwe and Mozambique (the Forbes Border Post), through which pass significant amounts of trade to and from the Mozambican port of Beira, on the southern Indian Ocean, not least of which is the Feruka pipeline which brings crude oil supplies from the Beira docks to Zimbabwe's oil refineries. Mutare is roughly equidistant between Harare (263km to the northwest) and Beira (290km east), and it was the establishment of the original rail link between the two that gave prominence, and form, to the town in 1897.

The town sits in a valley in the highlands that mark Zimbabwe's eastern border area. To the north the hills rise steeply to culminate in Mount Inyangani (the highest peak in the country) and the surrounding Nyanga area. To the south stand the heights of Bvumba, and further off Chimanimani. The valley has been the site of human occupation for a very long time. Hills surrounding the town contain San rock paintings,[2] and the ruins of Iron Age settlements. From at

[2]   The San/Khoi peoples were the original, indigenous inhabitants of southern Africa. Such rock paintings are variously dated at between 1000 and 2000 years old. Remnants of these peoples still survive in Namibia and southern

least the 15th century, the area has been settled by Manyika people, a Shona sub-group. Michael Bourdillon gives this account of the origins of Manyika settlement:

> One significant group from the Mutapa state travelled around the northeast corner of the plateau, settling beyond what are now the eastern highlands of Zimbabwe and subjecting the autochthonous Tonga to the rule of a new state. These people became known as the Barwe and their rulers were significant political figures in later dealings with the Portuguese. An offshoot from the Barwe state travelled eastwards onto the highlands and there founded the Chikanga dynasty of the Manyika peoples .... Originally the name Manyika applied only to the people around what is now Mutare, and the extension of the name to neighbouring peoples occurred through the influence of missionary activity and white government administration in the 20th century. The extension of the name is now accepted by the people themselves, who thereby acknowledge a certain unity between the chiefdoms so designated. (Bourdillon 1976: 18)

The term 'Shona' is now widely seen as a construct of British colonization. As late as the 1940s, the anthropologist J.F. Holleman feels the need, in the introduction to his magisterial *Shona Customary Law*, to explain his use of the term:

> The usefully inclusive, but foreign (Ndebele?) term 'Shona' will be used in describing the general pattern common to all communities in central Mashonaland because no other term seems to exist which could conveniently be used as a common denominator. (Holleman 1952: 2)

And, writing in 1976, Michael Bourdillon has this to say of the term 'Shona' when used as an ethnic classification:

> Now the peoples classified as 'Shona' cover most of Zimbabwe and parts of Mozambique, stretching to the Zambezi River in the north

[2] ctnd Angola. It is timely to recall this fact when, in Zimbabwe, the word 'indigenous' has become integral to the politics of exclusion, along with the decidedly odd phrase, 'son of the soil'.

and the Indian Ocean in the east. The derivation of the word 'Shona' is uncertain. It appears to have been used first by the Ndebele as a derogatory name for the people they had defeated, and particularly the Rozvi.[3] (op.cit: 17)

Bourdillon gives a detailed summary of pre-colonial Shona history, and the works of David Beach (1994, 1980) have been especially important in synthesizing what might be known about the history of preliterate peoples from a range of sources: oral histories, archival material (primarily Portuguese), and archeological exploration. Briefly, Bourdillon summarizes the matter thus:

> Shona history shows the rise and fall of a number of larger states, a long history of mining and a history of both internal and external trade. The Shona peoples had for the most part maintained their autonomy against various outside influences. (Ibid: 14)

Early colonists were attracted to the site by the existence of gold deposits at nearby Penhalonga. Indeed these gold sources had been exploited by local peoples prior to colonization, and had formed part of thriving trade links between the Mwene Mutapa dynasty (the kingdom which predated the Rozvi) and Portuguese traders from as early as the 15th century (Beech 1980). As a result the earliest colonial settlement was some 25km north-west of the city's current site, in a place now known as Old Mutare (and itself subsequently the site of an important Methodist mission, and now of Africa University), and was only moved at the time of the rail link in 1897. The town achieved status as a municipality in 1914. Originally known in colonial times as Umtali, the town reverted to its original Shona name of Mutare in 1981, after independence.

---

[3] 'The Shona did not call themselves by this name and at first disliked it; even now they tend rather to classify themselves by their chiefdoms or their dialect groups (Karanga, Manyika, Zezuru, Korekore, etc.), though most accept the designation Shona in contrast to unrelated peoples. The extension of the term to all tribes native to Zimbabwe appears to have been a British innovation.' M.F.C. Bourdillon 1976, 17.

Contemporary Mutare

The population of Mutare is probably in the region of 189,000 people (these figures come from the Zimbabwe Government Census of 2002). There are severe difficulties researchers now encounter in obtaining accurate statistical information on Zimbabwe and therefore, as with all other government sources, these figures should be treated with some skepticism.[4] However, some indication of the rapid growth of the town in the past two decades of post-colonial rule is to be found in a comparison of the 2002 figure with that from the 1982 census which estimated Mutare's population at just under 70,000. (Manicaland as a whole, of which Mutare is the provincial capital, is the second most densely populated province in Zimbabwe, after the Harare/Chitungwiza urban conglomerate, again according to the dubious figures of the 2002 Zimbabwe Government Census). Similar processes of rapid urbanization have been documented elsewhere in southern Africa.

Mutare covers an area of roughly 16,700 hectares. The patterns of settlement are similar to those found throughout Zimbabwe's urban areas (and, indeed, probably throughout southern Africa's ex-British colonies and protectorates). Under colonial rule urban land use was racially demarcated. In Mutare, the eastern side of the town, closest to the border with Mozambique, and nestled beneath the hills of Cecil Kop, are the larger plots (originally of one acre each) designated for white settlers. Further down in the valley, running roughly along the railway line and adjacent to the town's commercial district, are smaller plots originally designated for Asian and 'coloured' (mixed race) groups. These formed a barrier between 'white' areas

---

[4] Population figures, even prior to the last census of 2002, were unreliable. The situation has become even less clear since. In particular large displaced populations as a result of land reform (such as commercial farmworkers) and Operation Murambatsvina (the poor, urban underclass) are unaccounted for. See Hammar, McGregor and Landau 2010.

and, stretching away south-westwards, much smaller plots and more densely populated 'black townships'. Post-colonial rule has renamed these divisions as low density (previously white and middle class) and high density (previously black and working class). The racial divisions have fallen away, the class ones remain. Thus was class and colour mapped onto the landscape, with forms of the colonial inscription enduring on into current times.

In three decades of post-colonial rule, the city has seen rapid expansion, as we have seen indicated in official population figures. Most noticeably this has given rise to large-scale expansions of high-density areas. The original township of Sakubva has been added to by Dangamvura, Chikanga (phases 1 through 5), and Hobhouse (phases 1 and 2). The barracks of the Zimbabwe Army's Third Brigade have also been substantially redeveloped to include housing for officers and ordinary soldiers. Currently the city claims to have 15 primary schools (for children aged six through 12), 11 secondary schools (for children aged 13 through 18) and over 12 various tertiary education facilities (Africa University, which at the time of writing is the country's only functioning university, as well as three teacher training colleges, a polytechnic college and a variety of other vocational skills training centres, most noticeably in computer-related technology). Once again, the figures should be treated with caution. As the national education system has all but closed down there has been a boom in private colleges, which take the place of secondary schools. I know of no accurate figures either in regard to how many government schools are still functioning (and to what capacity), or in regard to how many 'new' private colleges have emerged to replace failed state secondary schools.[5]

[5] This paragraph on education reflected the situation in Mutare, during the time of my fieldwork, prior to the signing of the Global Political Agreement (GPA), which brought into being the Government of National Unity (GNU), in late 2008. One major accomplishment of the GNU has been the re-opening of schools and tertiary colleges. However, it remains true to my knowledge that

As with education and housing, so with health. Post-colonial Zimbabwe inherited an uneasy mix of public and private provision. Not all of the private provision is for the wealthy either. Some estimates are that up to 40% of national health and education facilities are provided by churches, especially in rural areas, most frequently in established missions run by the mainstream churches. Most people in Mutare have found healthcare at the Mutare General Hospital (officially the provincial hospital since it acted as a tertiary referral centre for the whole of Manicaland Province). I use the past tense here as the hospital has been in a very dire state for at least the past three years. I know of no reliable figures for the numbers of doctors, nurses and other technicians still working. (Media reports often state that the large Zimbabwean diaspora is substantially composed of professionals: doctors, nurses and teachers being the most numerous.)

However, accurate statistics are unavailable, although media reports often refer to the total Zimbabwean diaspora as numbering around three million, out of a total estimated national population of around 11 million at the time of the last National Census in 2002). There are very great shortages of basic medical supplies, including basic drugs. Standards of hygiene are parlous, to say the least. For most of 2008 the majority of people in the town believed the hospital to be closed; not entirely accurately, for as we shall see, the paediatric clinics were still functioning though probably at a greatly reduced capacity. The state Ministry of Health and the City's

5 ctnd there are no reliable statistics on schools, numbers of teachers (and their qualifications), or pass rates both at primary and secondary levels. In Mutare, the private colleges which flourished during the period of closure in the government schools continue to exist suggesting that families have yet to be convinced of the reliability of government educational provision for their children. Most recently, Amnesty International have released a report (October 2011) claiming that a quarter of a million Zimbabwean children experienced or continue to experience significant disruptions to the their education as a result of Operation Murambatsvina. See www.amnestyinternationalusa.org.

Department of Health itself also provide satellite clinics, both in the central business district and in at least three high-density locations. These provide basic medical care, often by very overworked nurses, and some maternity services. Again it is unclear how well staffed or well supplied such clinics are, or indeed to what extent they are still running.[6]

Historically, Mutare had an economy based on the supply and support services necessary for surrounding agricultural and mining ventures. Timber, fruit, tobacco, bananas, flowers, gold and diamonds have all played important roles in the local economy. A short drive through the town will reveal a wide variety of shops, wholesale and retail, selling farming and building supplies, machinery, spare parts and mechanics and all manner of other businesses supplying and supporting rural production. Inevitably, along with the rest of the country's economy, these businesses have suffered catastrophic losses as a consequence of chaotic land reform, hyperinflation, falling employment levels and general economic and political mismanagement. Up until the country abandoned its own worthless currency in January 2009, and adopted the US dollar and the South African rand, it was a very common sight to see supermarkets and warehouses entirely empty of goods.

Of churches and diamonds

There have been, in recent times, what we might term 'growth industries' in Mutare though. The first has come in the form of an explosive growth in Pentecostal Christian churches. This is, of course, a phenomenon widely noted throughout sub-Saharan Africa (and

[6]   Following the GPA of 2008, health institutions and services have also officially reopened. Again there are no reliable statistics for medical staff, resources, drug availabilities, etc. Costs are also prohibitive for poor, urban people. For example, a single visit to the Mutare hospital costs $6 (in a country where the vast majority of the population survives on less than $2 per day).

indeed many other parts of the global south) (Robbins 2004). Over the past four years, along one street in central Mutare I have counted the establishment of over five new churches, all in the vein of charismatic, Pentecostal worship. To pass along this street on a Sunday is to experience an extraordinary cacophony of song, ecstatic preaching, jubilation and intense sociality. These churches are also found throughout low- and middle-class areas of the city. They stand alongside, and compete actively with, the mainstream churches (which here I take to mean those churches that have been present in Zimbabwe for long periods of time: Roman Catholic, Anglican, Methodist, Presbyterian, Seventh Day Adventist and Baptist, to name but the most obvious). Newer churches tend not to belong to these older Christian groupings and to bear names such as The Lighthouse, the Embassy of Christ or Christian Fellowships, although the distinctions are often more blurred. Some of these churches are indigenous to Africa (Christ Embassy is a Nigerian-based church) or even indigenous to Zimbabwe (Zimbabwe Assemblies of God Africa, or ZAOGA, is a transnational evangelical movement well documented by David Maxwell, 2006).

The second source of intense economic and social growth within Mutare over the past four years has come from its proximity to the alluvial diamond fields near Chiadzwa, in Marange, approximately 30km away. The presence of significant deposits of high quality diamonds in the area had been known for some time, and various established companies had claimed stakes in their development. Commercial mining claims fell victim to the general confusion in Zimbabwe over the past decade with regard to property rights. In 2005 there was an explosion of shallow digging in the area by a wide range of people; some local to the area and others who had travelled some distance to make their fortunes. Very quickly networks of diggers and dealers were established. Mutare witnessed a sudden burst of new-found wealth: new and expensive cars were visible on the streets, house prices and sales showed a strong, sharp and sudden surge. It was a very visible form of wealth for a few, although there were also less profitable forms of economic opportunity suddenly available to others who would travel the short distance to sell food, beer and other supplies to diggers. For some months the bus stands serving Marange were sites of intense, 24-hour activity. As is now well known, the ruling party and its military allies moved in quickly to regain control of this sudden source of great wealth and the area and its wealth appears to have become the site of another blood diamond debacle involving mass death, abductions, and forced labour. The details have yet to be fully revealed. (See the reports of the Solidarity Peace Trust, for example.[7])

Diamonds and churches constitute the most obvious growth industries in contemporary Zimbabwe. There are others. Cheap Chinese domestic products, second-hand clothing markets and a very broad array of technology outlets (especially those concerned with cell phones) are also very evident.[8]

The borders of the Zimbabwean

A defining feature of Mutare is its proximity to the border with Mozambique. Michael Bourdillon has this to say of Zimbabwe's eastern border:

> One early consequence of colonial settlement was the drawing of the boundary between Portuguese East Africa and the British colony of Southern Rhodesia. This boundary was negotiated in Lisbon and London with little regard for the Shona peoples resident in border areas. The boundary sometimes separated related groups of Shona

---

[7] Access to, and accurate information on, mining activities at Chiadzwa and in other parts of Marange are now strictly controlled and extremely opaque. The history of the site and its wealth is in urgent need of further detailed study in its own right.

[8] This is a national phenomenon it would seem. Again see Jones 2010, and Mawowa and Matongo 2010.

and sometimes even went right through established chiefdoms.[9] (Bourdillon op.cit: 15)

The border (as is common with many colonial demarcations) follows geographical features (in this case, the foothills of the highlands) but bears no relation to populations and their cultural links. People on both sides of the border are Shona sub-groups, Manyika speaking in the north and Ndau in the south. The movement of people and goods also bears little relationship to borders. Many Mutare people will admit to having kin on the Mozambican side, and outside of urban spaces, paths over the border are numerous and well known. Indeed, until mid-2008, it was necessary for a Zimbabwean to have a visa to enter Mozambique. Both passports and visas were expensive and difficult to obtain. Mutare residents would, however, frequently joke about their (numerous) trips to Mozambican towns via 'the green route' (i.e. paths over the green hills). Despite wars (during some of which long stretches were mined) the border has remained porous to local peoples and largely resistant to official surveillance or attempts at control. One such path, well cleared and travelled began close to our house, and it was not an infrequent sight to see people passing over the hills, in both directions. Indeed the border has its own long history, entwined in local memory and lore. Among the people of the Tangwena chieftaincy, above Nyanga, whole populations followed their chief Rekai Tangwena into Mozambique during the later years of the Second Chimurenga.[10] This chapter of Zimbabwean his-

---

[9] 'Since Portuguese colonial policy differed from British policy, the Shona in Mozambique and in Zimbabwe found themselves subject to different and separate influences. The greater economic growth in Zimbabwe and the greater attention of Zimbabwe settlers in this country to the education of indigenous peoples resulted in growing cultural differences across the frontier. Now many recognize the frontier as being more significant than the traditional boundaries of ancient Shona states.' M.F.C. Bourdillon 1976, 15.

[10] 'Second Chimurenga' refers to the (valorized) guerilla war against the Smith-led settler regime (1965-1980) which led to independence and majority rule in 1980.

tory and its instantiations in current memory and expectation have been well documented by the anthropologist, Donald Moore in *Suffering for Territory* (2003).

The border with Mozambique, however, also marks the site of an 'other'. In previous decades it was the pitied, poorer neighbour and the source of refugees, fleeing the extended Mozambican civil war (itself funded by the Smith regime in Rhodesia, apartheid-era South Africa and Reagan-era America).[11] In an ironic reversal of fortune, the past decade has made the nearer towns of Mozambique (Manica and Chimoio) magnets for Zimbabwean shoppers (of all classes) who flock to (mostly South African owned) supermarkets and wholesalers. It has also become a site for Zimbabwean migrants to seek new lives. White Zimbabwean commercial farmers have become a particular category of obvious newcomers in these (and other) Mozambican towns (Hammar 2010). Mozambique represents the 'other' in darker ways too. People in Mutare have frequently told me, in conversations about traditional healers and witchcraft, that the most 'powerful' healers (and by implication witches) are to be found in Mozambique. 'Strong medicine' (*mushonga*) is to be found either over the border or in the 'deep rural areas'. Chipinge, a rural village some 300km south, is often cited as the only Zimbabwean area whose healers can rival the powers of those from Mozambique.

The Zimbabwean crisis and Mutare

One of the defining events for all Zimbabwean urban centres over the past decade has been the growth of the Movement for Democratic Change (MDC), the first serious political challenge to the hegemony of ZANU-PF since it came to power at independence in 1980. Fol-

[11] The Mozambican civil war, 1977-1992, pitted the FRELIMO Marxist government which took control after the end of Portuguese colonial rule in 1976 against an armed insurgency called RENAMO, funded by the US and SA, and widely seen by historians as a proxy conflict of the global Cold War.

lowing on from the political challenge, came a series of government crackdowns on urban populations (widely seen to be the bedrock of opposition support) which have included the erosion of local structures of political autonomy (elected town councillors and mayors), and direct displacements of the urban poor (most dramatically) in the form of Operation Murambatsvina (Clean Out the Trash). In Mutare, the days of the mass urban displacement was a time of burning. For most of a week we all watched a spiral of smoke rising above the city's poorer areas. High-density areas bore the brunt of the violence but, in the business district, long established vegetable and fruit markets were also affected. Goods were 'confiscated' (without compensation, i.e. stolen by the police), people beaten and well-established livelihoods destroyed.[12]

The dark days of Operation Murambatsvina marked my own entry into Mutare as a researcher. Originally, at the outset of this project in early 2005, I had intended to work with HIV-positive children in an established project in the sprawling squatter camp outside Harare, known as Hatcliffe Extension. By July 2005, Operation Murambatsvina had entirely destroyed those communities. I began preliminary explorations into relocating my study site to Mutare in March 2005 and had moved there completely by June. Zimbabwe had entered a deepening spiral of fear, and surveillance. Re-locating myself and my intended study to a smaller urban centre seemed sensible under the conditions, and a possible way of avoiding (or at least reducing) unwanted attention.

I entered the current research field first as a child psychotherapist, interested in establishing a 'psycho-social support group' for HIV-positive children. Similar groups have mushroomed in response to the needs of such children who are living in situations of poverty and adversity. Although widely represented as appropriate and effec-

[12] For more detail on Operation Murambatsvina and its consequences see the two reports by the Solidarity Peace Trust 2005, Hammar, McGregor and Landau 2010, and Musoni 2010.

tive ways in which institutions can respond to the needs of children, there is little firm evidence as to their effectiveness, and I was interested in both exploring the interventions further and using them as an entry point to direct contact with children living in extreme adversity. The current climate of fear and silence in Zimbabwe[13] brings with it a deep wariness of the stranger and my initial approaches to government and NGOs were greeted with hesitance, silence and avoidance. There was a long period of time (over three months) when the research was stalled and the periods of waiting for responses felt like tests of endurance, seriousness, authenticity and security.

Eventually a small NGO based in Mutare and concerned with orphans on surrounding commercial farms agreed to allow me to accompany them on a round of visits to the support groups they ran. The set of visits allowed me to meet a number of children and adult facilitators, and to observe the workings of the groups, which were largely activity based and income generating. They operated as clubs and focused on vegetable growing, sports and other activities such as drama, dance and gospel singing. It was unclear to me what was psy-

---

[13] This is clearly a generalization. Writing it, I was thinking of fear and silence as direct outcomes of the nationwide organized violence that has been a central feature of social life during the Zimbabwean crisis (which I would date from the defeat of the government in the constitutional referendum and the onset of 'land invasions' in 2000 and running through to today where, despite the GNU, there are many incidents of organized violence, particularly in the periods leading up to elections). However Zimbabweans can be said to have endured repeated waves of social violence and, therefore, of silence and fear over the past 100 years at least. See many of the contributors to Harold-Barry (2004), but especially Tony Reeler's essay in that volume. See also Raftoupolos and Savage (2004). It is useful here to recall Fanon's (1961) insistence that colonialism (and decolonization) were as much psychological as political, and intrinsically violent. For a more recent anthropological study of social violence and silence see Das 2007, and various contributors to the volume *Tense Past: cultural essays on trauma and memory*, edited by Paul Antze and Michael Lambek (1996). For current psychological perspectives on trauma and silence see the edited volume *Beyond Trauma: cultural and societal dynamics*. Kleber, Figley and Gersons, 1995.

chological about the activities although clearly they were very useful as forms of general support, income generation and peer bonding. What was most striking was the intense poverty under which the children lived, as the children of commercial farmworkers in the aftermath of the collapse of commercial farming in Zimbabwe as a consequence of sustained political assault. (The plight of commercial farmworkers and their dependents in the aftermath of the 'land reform' in Zimbabwe is a subject deserving of extensive study in its own right. See Blair Rutherford, 2001, for a useful analysis of their difficult lives prior to the demise of commercial farming.[14]) These children had almost no access to clinics or schools. One group of children I interviewed was enrolled at a rural school 25km away and it entailed a three-hour walk each way, often on one inadequate meal a day. The heroics of commitment to education under such circumstances have not been sufficiently recorded or extolled.

Subsequently, I managed to establish contact with two local paediatricians who had strong links with a large NGO that focused on supporting those living with the virus. I agreed to establish a group under their auspices for HIV-positive children as an exploration of their specific psychological and social needs and the ways in which a therapeutic group might provide a useful forum for elaborating and meeting these needs. The doctors agreed to refer children from their clinics at the local provincial hospital, and we agreed that the group would initially be for children aged between 12 and 18 years of age. Although there were yet further delays in starting the group (the doctors were slow to refer probably reflecting both their heavy workloads and their uncertainty about the usefulness of the group), some two months later, in November 2005, an initial eight children met

[14] In relation to displaced commercial farmworkers see also Kinsey (2010) and Magaramombe (2010). I do not think that the lives of commercial farmworkers can be generalized (prior to land reform). From the 1990s there is some evidence suggesting that, in certain areas, the children of farmworkers had better nutrition and schooling than other children in, for example, rural, peasant communities.

me for the first time. We have met weekly since for over four years.

Next I give descriptions of the children I have come to know through the group and whose lives form the bulk of the ethnography that follows.

The children in the group

I use the word 'children' throughout the study although, as will be noted, most of the children are what would now commonly be referred to as 'adolescents'. I do this for two reasons. Firstly, the concept of adolescence was developed in the context of a normative (western) trajectory of developmental psychology. As Erica Burman (2008) has shown, it is a common, and mistaken, assumption that such normative models can be applied to other socio-economic, cultural or gender contexts. Furthermore, it is now some 50 years since Philippe Aries (1962) demonstrated the interpellated histories of childhood, family and education in Western Europe. In his analysis, categories within childhood, and indeed childhood itself, arose in relationship to ideas about institutional education and the development of hierarchies of knowledge that came to be associated with age. Outside of the West, and particularly in Zimbabwe, where the education system has so conspicuously collapsed, it is unclear that the distinctions are meaningful. Secondly, as will become clear, many of the children are both stunted and underweight. They do not look like adolescents or young adults. Therefore the use of the term 'children' both de-centres certain western norms and serves to remind us of physical appearances and discrepancies.

Here I give details and brief descriptions of the children, all HIV-positive, whom I have come to know well through the auspices of the group. Informed consent was obtained from the children and their caretakers both to join to group and to be part of the ethnographic study (two separate processes). As noted above, the group began meeting in November 2005. It continues to meet weekly at the time of writing (April 2010[15]). The case material presented in my writing comes from the children of the group, and their caretakers. I have changed all names and identifying particulars in order to protect their confidentiality. There is no record, other than in my memory, of connections between the actual children and ways in which I have represented them here. The start of the group coincided roughly with the rollout of antiretroviral drug treatments (ARVs) in Mutare; hence many of the children began ARV treatment at about the same time, although almost all had previously been on the prophylactic antibiotic, cotrimoxazole.

Priscilla was 14 years old when I first met her in 2005. She was diagnosed HIV-positive at birth in a Harare hospital in 1991. Initially she lived with her mother and grandmother (mother's mother) in Harare. Her parents had begun the proceedings for a formal divorce before her father's death in 1996. Her mother, also known to be HIV-positive, died in 2001. Her grandmother (her principal caretaker) died in 2003. Since 2003, Priscilla has lived with her mother's sister in Mutare. She has an independent elder sister who lives in Harare, and a younger sister who lives with her maternal grandfather and his new wife in Bulawayo. Her aunt's household currently numbers ten people, living on two small salaries. They all share four rooms, which are rented in a high-density suburb. Her relationship with her aunt's husband is conflictual. He feels she should be cared for by her father's family. Priscilla is very underweight and looks at least five years younger than her chronological age. Her education has been sporadic. She has had at least two periods of noncompliance with ARVs, and at least one suicide attempt (when she drank domestic bleach in a small quantity). In addition she has been diagnosed with drug-resistant tuberculosis. Her health is very poor. Priscilla is now 19 years old and still in school when her health permits and money is available for fees.

[15] I am writing in the ethnographic present tense in these descriptions.

Susan was 13 years old when I first met her in 2005. She was diagnosed HIV-positive at birth in Mutare in 1992. She lived with her mother for the first year of her life. Her mother was known to be HIV-positive. Her parents were never married. Her father was already married and Susan has a half-sister of roughly her own age. Susan has lived with her father, her stepmother and her half-sister since infancy; she has close relationships with them all. The family lived in a rented house in a high-density suburb. She has no memories of her mother, who died when she was two years old. She does have regular contact with her mother's family. Her father is HIV-positive. He is an electrician and her stepmother is a nurse. Since 2008 her father has been resident in South Africa where he has a job. Susan's parents are well educated with two incomes. She has been on ARVs since 2006 (as has her father) and her adherence has been good. Her health is good, with age appropriate height and weight. Her school attendance and achievement are both good. In late 2009 Susan and the rest of her family relocated to South Africa to join her father. Susan is now 18 years old, and seeking a place in a college for tertiary education.

Kuda was 15 years old when I first met her in 2006. She too was diagnosed HIV-positive at birth in Mutare in 1989. Both her parents are dead (her father died in 1991 and her mother in 1994). She has lived with her aunt (her mother's sister) since prior to her parents' death. There are five people in the household that comprises of two adults and three children. Her aunt and uncle own a small butchery and bottle store, as well as the small house in a high-density suburb in which they live. Kuda has been on ARVs since 2008 and her adherence is good. Her health is good as are her height and weight. She has a reputation in her neighbourhood as a gifted hairdresser and would like to obtain a formal qualification but the family is currently unable to afford the fees. Kuda is now 20 years old.

Matilda was 11 years old when I met her in 2006. She was diagnosed HIV-positive at birth in Marondera in 1995. When I met her she had recently moved to Mutare to stay with her father's sister. Previously she had stayed in two different households (her mother's sister and her mother's brother). Her father died in 1998. Her mother was also dead but I do not know when she died. She had two siblings (a brother of 14 and a sister of 17) at the time of our meeting. She began taking ARVs in 2006. Her health was poor. She was stunted and underweight and looked at least three years younger than her age. Her schooling had been very sporadic. Matilda was very shy and inarticulate. Her attendance at the group was also very sporadic. The family of her father's sister consisted of two adults and their four children who lived in a rented house in a high-density suburb. Her aunt was a teacher. In 2008 Matilda was sent to stay with her sister. In 2009 I received news that she had died earlier that year.

Thandi was seven years old when I met her in 2008. She was diagnosed HIV-positive at birth in 1997 in Mutare. Her mother is also HIV-positive and the two live together, in two rented rooms in a high-density suburb. They have no contact with Thandi's father or his family, who dispute his paternity on the grounds that he claims he does not have HIV. Thandi's mother is a local HIV activist; however her income comes primarily from her work selling vegetables in one of the street markets. Both mother and daughter have been on ARVs since 2006. Thandi is healthy. Her mother is blind in one eye after a bout of HIV-related herpes zoster. Thandi attends school. She is now 14 years old.

Damiso was an 11-year-old boy when I met him in 2005. He was born in Mutare in 1994, and diagnosed shortly after birth as HIV-positive. Both his parents died before 1998. His five elder brothers, all of whom are young adults, have been his primary caretakers. At the time that I met him he was staying with his oldest brother's wife's sister in a very poor neighbourhood. All his brothers had moved to South Africa. He is related to Thandi's mother through the marriage of one of his brothers. He had commenced ARVs in 2006. He was stunted and underweight appearing, to be some years younger than his actual age. His health was generally poor although the ARVs did seem to steadily improve his susceptibility to infection. His relationship with his caretaker was poor and her care of him negligible. He was in school. In 2008, he left for South Africa to join his brothers. I have heard he is doing well there.

Persistence was a 12-year-old boy when I met him in 2006. He was born in the rural area of Makoni South in 1994, and diagnosed in 1996 as HIV-positive. He lived with his mother and younger brother in two rooms in a high-density suburb of Mutare. One of his mother's sisters and her two children lived in an adjoining two rooms. His mother was HIV-positive. His father died in 1998. His mother and her sister support themselves and their children through selling vegetables in a street market. In addition, his mother is an occasional 'cross-border' trader (someone who crosses to neighbouring countries to purchase small, domestic goods for resale). Persistence began taking ARVs in 2006. He was underweight and stunted, and appeared at least three years younger than he is. Despite his poor health he had done generally well in school. Persistence died in late 2008, probably as a result of complications arising from a bout of malaria. His younger brother Kudzi subsequently joined the group and is now 14 years old. He has been on ARVs since 2008, helps his mother in the market and is a remarkably good student.

Takura was an 11-year-old boy when I met him in 2006. He was born in Mutare in 1995 and diagnosed HIV-positive around that time. He lives with his mother and younger brother in two rented rooms in a high-density suburb. His mother supports the family through work in a street market and other itinerant work (e.g. grass cutting for the municipality). He has been on ARVs since 2006 and his health has improved although he is still small and underweight for his age. His father died in 2001. His mother was subsequently disowned and dispossessed by her late husband's family. There is no contact between the boys and their father's family. Takura's younger brother and his mother are also HIV-positive. His mother is on

ARVs. His younger brother is not and is much healthier and stronger than Takura. He is in school and is now 16 years old.

Tinashe was 10 years old when I met him in 2005. He was born in Mutare in 1995 and diagnosed HIV-positive at that time. His mother is also HIV-positive. He has a three-year-old half-brother, who is also HIV-positive (with a different father who is no longer around). Tinashe's father died in 1998. He has close relationships with his father's family, especially his grandmother (his father's mother) who live in Zimunya, a rural area some 30km from the city. Tinashe lives with his mother and younger brother in two rented rooms in a high-density suburb. His mother supports the family by brewing and selling beer although she sometimes also practices cross-border trading. Tinashe has had a difficult relationship with his mother and has often spent extended periods staying with his grandmother. The moves between households have meant severe disruption to his schooling. His health is poor; he is underweight and stunted. He has also suffered extensively from severe skin rashes over most of his body with secondary infections. His eyesight is poor. He has been on ARVs since 2006, as has his mother. He is now 15 years old.

Stephen was 12 years old when I met him in 2005. He was born in Zimunya, a rural area outside Mutare in 1993, and diagnosed HIV-positive shortly after. His mother died in 1994 and his father in 1995. He lived with his grandmother (his mother's mother) on the outskirts of a high-density suburb in a makeshift shack. His grandmother lived in great poverty, doing some market work and being helped by her neighbours. He had an older brother aged about 17 whose whereabouts were unknown to his grandmother. Stephen's health was very poor. He was stunted and severely underweight. He began taking ARVs in 2005. He was very close to his grandmother and disliked talking to others. He died three months after the start of our group.

Nicholas was a 16-year-old boy I met in 2007 who had recently been diagnosed HIV-positive. He attributed this to his recent sexual activity. He was commenced on ARVs shortly after his diagnosis. He was still in school and lived with his father and his stepmother in a small rented house in one of the city's oldest high-density areas. He had two younger siblings. I do not know the HIV status of the other members of the family. His illness was a source of embarrassment and shame to his family, which was something that caused him great shame and sorrow. He died in early 2009.

Isaiah was 15 years old when I met him in 2005. He was born in Mutare in 1990, the youngest of four boys. His mother died in 1993 and his father in 1996. Isaiah lives with his grandmother (his father's mother) in one rented room in a high-density suburb. He was diagnosed HIV-positive shortly after birth. He has been on ARVs since 2006. He has a severe hearing deficit probably as a result of repeated ear infections in early childhood. Partly as a result his education has been poor and his social skills underdeveloped. He supports himself and his grandmother by itinerant work in street markets, although they also receive some help from one of his aunts. His health is poor and he is very underweight. He has drug-resistant tuberculosis. Isaiah's elder brothers are sometimes in the household but appear to live peripatetic lives. They drink heavily according to their grandmother. I do not know their HIV status. Isaiah is now 20 years old.

In summary, I have come to know 13 children through the activities of the group. Five are girls, and eight are boys. All are cared for within their families although six have lost both parents. With the exception of Susan, all of their families live in varying degrees of severe poverty. All are now on ARVs and receive their medical care through the Mutare General Hospital's paediatric clinics. All but Nicholas are known to have been HIV-positive since infancy. Three children have died since the start of the group meetings, and three are in critically poor health as I write. My purpose here has been to give the reader outlines of the children in the group. More details follow as I use examples of children's lives and words in the chapters to follow.

Methodologies

The following is an account of the specific methodologies I used in the course of the fieldwork. This began, as noted above, with preliminary enquiries in March 2005 after my initial field site in a Harare shantytown was rendered impossible by an increased police presence. This was due to nationwide state-sponsored violence against the urban poor, referred to as Operation Murambatsvina, which took place between May and July 2005.

Between June and August 2005, I spent time meeting with NGOs said to be involved with children infected with HIV in and around urban Mutare. I began a support group under the auspices of the local paediatric clinic. It began meeting in November 2005 and constitutes the central element in my fieldwork. The size of the group has fluctuated between eight and 12 children, as some have died, others moved away and new children joined. I have paid transport costs for the children to attend and often provided food at the meetings. From 2007, the local Pentecostal church has been very helpful in providing the food for meetings. I have taken on other financial obligations in relation to all the children: help with the provision of food at home, as well as school and medical fees. I continue to give such support wherever possible. I have also assisted with funeral costs for children who have died.

Initially the group met at the offices of Family Aids Caring Trust (FACT), a local NGO with offices near the centre of town and the general hospital. The group met from 2 p.m. to 4 p.m. on Friday afternoons, a time that did not conflict with school hours. In April 2006, I moved the group meetings to a local church at the request of the children who were uncomfortable being seen going into the premises of an NGO known to be solely concerned with people living with HIV. The meeting times remained the same. We have continued to meet at the same venue since then. The group was for the children, and has been increasingly led and facilitated by them since its inception, although initially (for about the first four months) I took a lead. As the children have grown more confident in their own facilitation of group activities, I have withdrawn from a leadership role while still continuing to be present whenever I have been in Mutare. Typically, children have chosen to use the time to have conversations, play games, perform dramas and sing hymns. The material on which they base these activities tends to have been drawn from similar activities they have been involved in at school, in their neighbourhoods or in their churches. Wherever possible I have remained an observer. I have understood my own primary role as being one of developing relationships with the children and their caretakers. I did not attempt any probing, investigative conversations with children or their caretakers until I judged that I had established relationships of trust with them and that that trust had been rooted in my demonstrating a long-term commitment to them as individuals and as a group.

Often children are accompanied to meetings by caretakers. Like me, these adults are bystanders and our peripheral presence on the margins of the group has become a useful forum for further discussion and the development of relationships between them and me, and between themselves. I did not attempt any visits to children's homes until I had been invited and I did not request such invitations. Having been invited, I did begin to visit and subsequently became a regular visitor in most homes. I judged that such restraint was necessary both as a basic act of respect and out of a concern that children and their families should control my visits given that the visits of a white researcher would be noted by their communities at a time of both persistent stigma in relation to HIV and political fear and anxiety. In late 2008 and early 2009 I made a series of visits to all homes, with an assistant (a woman known to all from the church) in order to conduct detailed interviews about family histories, household compositions and incomes, illness experiences, religious beliefs and practices, and so forth. I believe that the interviews were remarkably detailed as a direct consequence of the solid relationships of trust that preceded them and on which they were therefore based. In addition, and once again only by invitation, I have accompanied children to functions at churches, schools and neighbourhood events. It should also be remembered that Mutare is a small town and that, therefore, I have often also met the children and their families in shops, markets, churches, and on roadsides.

I have also undertaken other forms of observation in order to better understand and contextualize the material I have been given by children and their families. With the generous permission and assistance of the paediatric staff at Mutare General Hospital, I carried out two periods of observing paediatric clinics – between January and February 2006, and again in December 2008 and January 2009. In both periods I attended the Wednesday morning clinic of a paediatrician that ran from 9 a.m. until the last patient had been seen, typically around noon. I then joined the doctor in his consulting room and was permitted to observe all his patient consultations. He was also kind enough to answer my many questions and to educate me in the medical issues and conditions he was diagnosing and treating, as well as to share with me the methodologies and outcomes of his own extensive research – over 25 years as a consultant in the institution. My engagement also allowed me to get to know the nursing staff and the procedures through which they administered the paediatric clinic as well as to observe the general bureaucracy of the hospital and the social forms of the waiting room.

As we shall see later in the ethnography, modern (western) medical practice sits alongside older forms of traditional healing. To explore these realms I met four traditional healers (n'angas) who practiced in Mutare. One of these was a prophet in the tradition of the African Independent Churches. I conducted interviews with these healers, and one of them generously allowed me to observe him consulting with patients for two days in October 2008. In addition I explored knowledge of healing herbs amongst the children and their caretakers.

The importance of Christian belief and practice, church membership and ideas about miraculous healing became increasingly apparent to me during the course of my fieldwork. From 2007 I began to attend a range of Christian churches in Mutare in order to observe ritual practice and to hear what teaching was offered in sermons, publications and so on. I was particularly interested in whether HIV-related illness was specifically addressed and the degrees to which children were incorporated into services. In the course of my attendances I met with a range of church leaders who had specific interests in children and HIV. The group included two Protestant pastors, two Catholic nuns and three other lay members who were all kind enough to agree to be interviewed and to share with me their views on HIV-positive children and their needs. Through my relationships with children and their families I was also present at healing services and funerals.

Additional fieldwork included interviewing teachers and pharmacists and closely monitoring local media reports. Finally, as with any anthropological fieldwork, I tried to remain very alert to local conditions and events, economic pressures and any other factors (local or national) that had relevance to my own direct range of concerns.

Observation has clearly been central to my ethnographic practice. By observation I mean a sustained, non-intrusive watching of the ways people behave and the contexts in which they do so. Such forms of observation are also central to many forms of psychotherapy. Observing the ways in which people behave often provides, in my experience, an interesting counterpoint to attention to what they say (which is also central to my work). For example, caretakers (especially mothers) may portray their relationships with their sick children in ways that approximate their ideals about how behaviour should be given the age of a particular child. However, it was frequently my observation that alerted me to behaviours that suggested more regressed, painfully tender interactions between children and adults. As we shall see, a dying 14-year-old boy (small and slight for his age) was put on his mother's back, in a manner common for infants, when he was at his weakest. Observation captured the behaviour of children in group process as well as with family members. These more protected interactions were often different to their behaviour in public spaces.

The psychotherapist and the ethnographer

I approached the task of facilitating the group (and, more generally, of building relationships with children and their families) primarily in the mode of the therapist: tolerating silence, encouraging talk on painful issues, being actively curious about their grief and joy, and avoiding concrete activities that might distract from these other tasks. It has, however, hardly been a therapeutic group in the classically accepted sense of the term. We began, for instance, meeting in a large room at the NGO's headquarters, which is primarily used as a storage room. The organization has strong Christian values and the walls are covered with a variety of posters: 'AIDS: there is no cure'and 'Spilt water cannot be recovered. The same applies to your virginity. Once lost it cannot be recovered. Guard it jealously!' We sat under the signs of a stern morality, much concerned with that which is lost, through foolishness and immorality, and cannot be reclaimed.

Indeed, the mode of the classical psychotherapist is itself oddly placed in these circumstances. On our first meeting, only one of the children openly admitted to having HIV, the others murmured of tuberculosis, or stomach infections. Furthermore, western forms of psychotherapy must also be understood as forms of institutional discourse with their own preferred forms and practices. The expression of feelings, the narrative mode and the notion of 'the self' are amongst these. It is entirely unclear that any of this holds much traction in Zimbabwean experiences of childhood and domesticity, and this study hopes to elucidate these issues further. However, this is a point at which to mark the wideness of the gap that may exist here. Consider the following description of traditional and rural accounts of the worlds of children amongst the Shona sub-group, the Karanga (who are geographical neighbours of the Manyika, to the southwest), taken from Herbert Aschwanden's ethnography:

> Future events are seen directly in children's dreams. If a child dreams that its grandmother is dead, it means that she will die within days or weeks. Children tell the truth, directly and bluntly, and their dream world is thought to be structured likewise. One stops children from telling their dreams for two reasons: the direct and probably correct message of the child's dream is much too 'shocking' for an adult. It is said that such dreams nip in the bud any doubts, and instead of taking defensive measures one resigns oneself to hopelessness. The second reason is as important: children frequently do not relate their own dreams correctly, so that a real recognition of the truth is doubtful …. The child itself is like a dream, the Karanga explain. Nobody knows what it thinks and how it has knowledge about many things which not even adults have. The child is a mystery to the Karanga. Children sometimes exhibit a relationship and a closeness to things in their environment which might 'shock' adults. For example, one watched children playing, in great harmony, with a poisonous snake. 'Shocked', the adult will kill the snake. But, it is said, this demonstrates that children live as in a dream. (Aschwanden, 1989: 272-3.)

In this extraordinary passage, there is a view of children, of the power of words and the nature of dreams that is quite radically different from that we receive from western psychology and psychotherapy and, in particular, from the deeply influential work of Sigmund Freud and his various and diverse followers. The difference marks some of the terrain needed to be covered in our attention to the life, worlds and expressions of children growing up HIV-positive in eastern Zimbabwe.

To return to my description of the early meetings of the group, and the origins of the ethnography, other painful paradoxes have included the fact that we often had to sit on sacks of maize meal and beans, food aid intended for others; an incongruity not lost on eight chronically hungry children and one discomforted therapist. One boy said, 'When people see me coming here every week they say I must have AIDS but I try to say that I'm only coming here because my aunt works here.' The church building does not carry that stigma although, in matters of piled food aid and stern moral messages, it is little different. I have become far less the detached therapist, providing an evenly hovering attention within the clear boundaries of the analytic hour and the rigorous formalities of personal distance and scrupulous payment. I have crossed the classical ethnographic and psychoanalytic boundary of the cool observer. The therapist, while still awkwardly present, has also become an advocate in pursuit of the ethnographic.

I hope to write more fully elsewhere about the therapeutic group processes at stake in the work. I believe the children benefited enormously from being a part of the peer group (which we might also call a 'psychosocial support group'). Such benefits included a safe space in which to discuss the dilemmas inherent in being HIV-positive, not least of which was the wholly new experience of being able to talk openly about their sero status. This was a slow process reliant on children coming slowly to positions of being able to trust each other. Thereafter children developed friendships that extended beyond the confines of the group, in its designated times and location. Some children lived in the same neighbourhoods or went occasionally to the same schools or churches. In a small town they met each other during the course of the day. It became increasingly common for me to hear the children recount incidents in which they had voluntarily met up in one or other outside context. As we shall see, I also began to hear of incidents in which they had come to each other's rescue in situations of social difficulty (when being taunted at school, when afraid to walk alone, when puzzled or hurt by social events which had occurred).

Positioning myself as the ethnographer

A description of the ethnography, however, would not be complete without some discussion of the effects of the work on me. It is recognized to be in the nature of ethnography, often described as a sustained engagement with others, that the ethnographer is increasingly implicated in the emotional and social worlds she is describing and attempting to understand. Friendships are formed, antipathies developed, relationships sustained and lost, and the flow of the self in the social followed and recorded. This is, however, a study of children living with life-threatening illness under conditions of dire poverty. Elsewhere I have described this as living under conditions of 'everyday extremity' (Parsons 2005): a grief-saturated and suffering social world where the most basic necessities of life must be fought for on a daily basis. In that paper, written at the outset of this work, I acknowledged that ethnography, like psychotherapy, implied the making of relationships with others which persist on in time and are not ultimately in the control of the researcher to end when the research ends. This, I imply, may be especially the case when the ethnographer is 'at home' and thus unable to finalise relationships with informants by leaving. Indeed the suffering informant elicits a complex web of emotions, a countertransference within the ethnography. Then I wrote:

> A true account of suffering, one that acknowledges both destruction and resilience, requires attention too to that which is in danger of being hidden, either through being subsumed by other pressing realities or because it elicits from us fear and denial of emotional pain. (Parsons 2005: 77)

I am at pains in what follows to be alert to the emotions I have felt that are inherent to this study: grief, guilt, anger, avoidance and denial (to name but a few of the most obvious). There have been other attempts in anthropology to attempt something similar. In his 'anthropology of decline' on the drastic and painful impoverishment of urban people living on the Zambian Copperbelt, James Ferguson (1999) wrote:

> The tragic course that so many people's lives were taking was not only an anthropological fact of some interest; it raised ethical and methodological difficulties of a sort that I was not well prepared to deal with. My fieldwork left me with a terrible sense of sadness, and a recognition of the profound inability of scholarship to address the sorts of demands that people brought to me every day in my research, as they asked me to help them with their pressing and sometimes overwhelming personal problems and material needs. I could proceed [with this book] only after arriving at the realization that decline, confusion, fear, and suffering were central subjects [of the book], and not mere background to it. (Ferguson 1999: 18)

Social change and the neglect of ordinary people

I have gestured towards ways in which I believe my training, and trained perceptions, as a psychotherapist were highly instrumental in initiating this study. It is an irony worth noting that my entry into the field as an ethnographer was greatly facilitated by my being a Zimbabwean (I did not need to apply for any form of study visa, or otherwise undergo any form of official scrutiny in embarking on the study), and by my being a psychotherapist, with specific skills in working with children and families. Prior to this work I had had quite extensive involvement in therapeutic work with victims of political violence and torture (see Parsons 2006; Parsons, Farrell and Frangoulis 2003), which was a form of professional work subject to intense official scrutiny and surveillance. By contrast, and I think as some form of a paradoxical gift, work with those infected with HIV appeared to be entirely without controversy. It appeared to elicit no official interest at all. This is a surprise to me since the failure of the Zimbabwean health system might well be taken as one of the more notable and obvious ways in which the post-colonial government has, conspicuously and egregiously, failed its own citizens. This point has been most forcefully made by Physicians for Human Rights, who have even suggested that the matter of the failed health system, and those responsible for its failure, be referred to the International Criminal Court in The Hague. The following is an extract from the summary of their very thorough report:

> The UN General Assembly, at its 2005 World Summit, has affirmed the principle of the Responsibility to Protect. At this summit, attended by over 170 member states, the member states acknowledged the necessity of intervening against the sovereignty of a State (under the UN Charter Chapter VII: Action with respect to threats to the peace, breaches of the peace, and acts of aggression) in order to protect the population of that State from state-sanctioned or state-permitted atrocities, including crimes against humanity. It is relevant to note that the UN Security Council has already stated that, unchecked, the HIV/AIDS pandemic may pose a risk to international stability and security. The epidemics of HIV/AIDS, cholera and TB currently raging in Zimbabwe pose threats to international peace and security in the region and beyond. Health services and essential aspects of public health infrastructure in Zimbabwe are now in a state of complete collapse. The policies and practices of the Mugabe regime precipitated the crisis, and the regime lacks the capacity, let alone the intent, to reverse it even with the support of the international agencies now providing emergency assistance. The Government has failed to engage in political and economic reforms necessary to enable health systems to recover. It has also obstructed the distribution of humanitarian aid. Only through the intervention of the international community can hospitals and clinics be reopened, supplies and drugs obtained, staff paid, and public health infrastructure be restored, so that the acute health care needs of the people of Zimbabwe can be met. Accordingly, the government of Zimbabwe should yield control

of its health services, water supply, sanitation, disease surveillance, Ministry of Health operations and other public health functions to a United Nations-designated agency or consortium. Such a mechanism would be equivalent to putting the health system into a receivership pursuant to the existence of a circumstance that meets the criteria for the Responsibility to Protect. This entity, taking full advantage of the human resources for health available in Zimbabwe (including administrative resources at the Ministry of Health), and generously supported by international donors, should assume all administrative responsibility for the operation of health services, water supply, sanitation and other public health functions until such time as a government capable of providing these services is in place. (Physicians for Human Rights 2009)

I quote a small part of the report at some length here in order to convey, in yet another way, the severity of the crisis in Zimbabwe, and the real effects of that crisis on healthcare. It is the convergence of a health system (and a country) in absolute crisis that frames the ethnography of children growing up HIV-positive in a small Zimbabwean town. The convergence can only lead to tragedy: for the children, for the town, for the ethnographer. Hence my title for the chapter: 'In this vale of tears', for this is a valley alive to Christian resonances of suffering as the lot of those on earth who come after The Fall, 'An ethnography of suffering and sorrow'; for the tragedy has been the object of study, the required point of attention and the events that I have not been able to avoid.

Ethics, grief and research

As previously stated, I have been very deeply moved in my relationships with the children and their families. This emotional attachment has grown over the course of what is now an extended engagement with a group of people over five years. I have watched children grow, and too often I have watched them die. For me, this writing cannot but resound with a continual sense of grief and loss. Indeed I take it as a measure of my success, and of the integrity and authenticity of the research that it represents, whether I can convey these losses to the reader.

There have been many times when I have experienced the work as an intense ethical burden.[16] Ethical dilemmas have arisen in relation to my work with the children and their families in a variety of ways. First among these, as I have already indicated, has been in relation to my felt need to provide materially for their needs whenever possible. I think that it is a feeling that I have imposed on myself more than it being the case that the children or their carers were demanding of me. It took me sometime to realize this.

I experienced my contacts with them as being demanded upon. I spent a great deal of time looking for money with which to provide them. I took this from my own research funds, from my friends, from business people I knew (and who I knew to be sympathetic to my work and to the needs of the children). I approached various NGOs on their behalf. The work of looking for money became very time-consuming and throughout the course of the study remained one of the main ways in which I occupied myself. I understand this as being both recognition of the extreme nature of their needs, and a repetition of an old pattern of colonial, paternalistic responsibility. In either case I felt it, in some profound way, my ethical responsibility to do all that I could to ensure that the children's basic needs were met. Such needs included food, medicines, school fees and clothing. There were of course many times when I was unable to provide anything. Such weeks were ones that distressed me. I would dread my meetings with the children, being empty-handed. I would find myself delaying leaving for meetings, inventing errands that would distract me. One of the workers at the church, Aunty Thandi (whom we shall hear from often in the course of the study, a prime inform-

---

[16] See my earlier paper on the extreme suffering of Zimbabwean children and the ethics of research, Parsons 2005.

ant) noticed my distress on one such day. 'You know,' she said, 'it is more important to them that you come, and talk to them, and remember their names and problems, than that you bring things.' At the time I was unconvinced, but touched by her concern and her attempt to comfort me, but now I think differently. What was at stake here was as much relationships as sources of material support. Both were desperately needed and sought after.

Another powerful way in which I have experienced the work as an ethical burden emerges more clearly now as I write and I think of it as a burden of representation. I am very concerned that I should do justice to the stories that were told me, to the lives and deaths that I witnessed. In this regard I understand 'doing justice' as writing the fullest account possible, providing the clearest description I can, and honouring that which I have witnessed in any way that seems possible in my writing of the study. At times I am haunted by the sense that I might be accused of making intellectual capital from the suffering of others, and a fulsome witness seems the only possible defence against such accusations. I need hardly add that I am my own chief accuser. 'Haunting', indeed, seems an apt word for my relationship to much of the material recounted here, for the vale of tears, despite its beauty, is a place of ghosts and the production of an ethnography of suffering and sorrow comes at a heavy price, of which I pay the least part.

3

Who cares?
Family, kin and other forms of caring

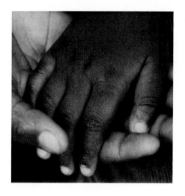

Introduction

Now I turn to what is perhaps one of the most basic and primary elements in the lives of children in Mutare who are growing up HIV-positive: their families, and those groups of relatives and friends who provide them with care, material and emotional. As we have seen from the previous chapters, children (like other vulnerable social groups) have been especially affected by the Zimbabwean crisis (now at least a decade old and showing few signs of resolving). I have described the place and form that the ethnography took, and the group of children I have come to know particularly well. I have also described the methods I used in conducting the ethnography.

My purpose here is to render as precisely and comprehensively as possible the quality of children's experiences of daily care within shifting, often transient care arrangements. Children both receive and offer care within shifting domestic terrains (although, of course, we are more usually attuned to the care they receive). The care, labour and support that children offer their families and their households have long been noted in anthropological and historical work on southern Africa. I do not imply newness here but, perhaps, a changing sharpness of emphasis. I also wish to highlight the ways in which the agentive work of children within the domestic realm, while hardly new in the scholarly literatures, profoundly challenges current 'global' ideas about child rights, appropriate child-rearing practices and the mental wellbeing of the young.

All of the children I know well are Shona, although not all of them would say that they are Manyika. It has been my experience that in urban areas children are always able and willing to tell you their regional Shona group membership (and clan) but these are often mixed. Sometimes children have described their parents as being 'mixed marriages', meaning alliances between people who would otherwise identify as Manyika, Zezuru, or Ndau, for example. While they may inhabit domestic worlds that appear fragile from the out-side, all the children I know express strong and clear ideas about the character of their families, including ideas about who belongs as a member of their family, what the rights and duties of members are, who holds authority and who requires what forms of respect. Indeed, children I know have very clear ideas about how respect should be performed and to whom.

Writing in the introduction to his *Growing up in Shona Society*, Michael Gelfand had this to say about his observations of Shona children over 30 years of fieldwork in a variety of Zimbabwean rural and urban spaces:

> Having been to Shona villages frequently over the years I found the customary way of bringing up a child most fascinating. The pleasant behavior of the child right up to adolescence stood out vividly. I have often envied this aspect of Shona society for, besides behaving well, the children seem happy. (Gelfand 1979: 2)

Gelfand's remark implies histories of closely intertwined theories of kinship and political economy, constituted by the colonial histories that framed them. As Peter Pels has noted in his analysis of the relationships over time between anthropology and colonialism:

> For anthropologists, more than for any other type of scholar, colonialism is not a historical object that remains external to the observer. The discipline descends from and is still struggling with techniques of observation and control that emerged from the colonial dialectic of Western governmentality. (Pels 1997: 164)

It is to the relationships between anthropological kinship theory and the political economies of colonialism in southern Africa that I turn next.

Kinship theory and colonial history in Southern Rhodesia

In this chapter I explore the children's felt experiences of familial and kinship care. I point this out since, as we shall see, the definition and classification of kinship systems is one of the most privileged sites of intense and lengthy debate within anthropology as a discipline, and we shall need to explore some of this technical literature in thinking about how families respond to domestic crisis and demand in contemporary Mutare, and in relation to the care of the sick and the young. The professional anthropological literature on kinship in Africa originated in the context of colonial power relations (Pels 1997), and we have seen in the previous chapter how the conditions of colonialism had both defined the Shona peoples as an ethnic group and demarcated (and truncated) the territory in which they lived.

The earliest substantial account of Shona kinship comes in the work of J.F. Holleman (1952). Holleman was a Dutch anthropologist, previously a student of both Radcliffe-Brown and Schapera. His intellectual ties spanned both the early functionalism associated with the British School of Malinowski and Radcliffe-Brown, and the *volkkundige* ('folk art') approach closely associated with German traditions of philologically-informed ethnology of Afrikaans anthropology, rooted at Stellenbosch in the Western Cape. Afrikaner anthropology subsequently gained a more sinister reputation through its active engagement with the intellectual formulations that would attempt to uphold apartheid; however, earlier in the 20th century, it was more involved with the recuperation of Afrikaner identity in the wake of British aggression and atrocities in the course of the two Boer wars.

Holleman's work in Southern Rhodesia, amongst the Hera Shona sub-group, was part of his engagement with the Rhodes-Livingstone Institute (RLI) (as a Beit Fellow) and, indeed, his field site was chosen for him by Max Gluckman, in keeping with the wide range of the Institute's regional research aims. Holleman's relationship with the intense, and intensely British, internal dynamics of the RLI, and its later manifestation as the Manchester School, was to prove difficult. Both Richard Werbner (1984) and Lyn Schumaker (2001), two important historians of the RLI, portray Holleman as an ethnographer who was significantly closer to colonial administrators and local white settlers than his more critically distanced colleagues at the Institute. Both historians portray him as isolated within the close ranks of the RLI, and as largely left to his own devices. Later on in his career, he would be a direct employee of the settler colonial government of Southern Rhodesia, although his major work, *Chief, Council and Commissioner* (1969), a subtle account of the complexities of local government under settler colonial political authority, I think, defies easy political categorization.

Holleman's fieldwork began in the mid-1940s when British colonial domination in Southern Rhodesia was fully engaged with the postwar politics of expansion, instantiated in continuing restrictions on 'native' access and entitlement to land, and on codifications of 'native law' (see Alois Mlambo, 2009 for a fuller account and for an interesting reflection on parallels between colonial policy in Southern Rhodesia and the 'new' Nationalist agenda in South Africa). With this proviso in our minds let us examine Holleman's account of Shona kinship.

All anthropological sources on Shona peoples are agreed that the basic system is patrilineal; this is to say that descent is traced through fathers' families, and fathers' family names. Holleman gives a lengthy account of Shona kinship systems from which I take the following:

> The basic genealogical unit is the exogamous, patrilineal clan, *rudzi*, a widely scattered body of people sharing the same clan name (*mutupo*) and the same 'sub-clan' name (*chidawo*). Clan names are, as a rule, of totemic origin, sub-clan names are not. (Holleman 1952: 23)

In Mutare, and more widely among the Manyika, the most common clan totems (plural: *mitupo*) are *shoko*/monkey and *shumba*/lion. The clan is exogamous, meaning that you may not marry (or have sexual relations) with anyone from the same clan totem as yourself, although they constitute large groups of people who may have no other social connection or knowledge of one another. To break the totem taboo is to break the incest taboo. The implication of the system is that, were one able to trace each totem group back far enough, one would come upon common patrilineal ancestors, the founders of the original totem:

> The main significance of the *rudzi* (clan) lies in the fact that on the strength of a common *mutupo* and *chidawo*, people claim a common origin through a patriline even when actual kinship cannot be traced, and that, the clan being exogamous, intermarriage between members is forbidden in principle. But even this rule is breaking down in some cases where actual relationship between the parties can no longer be traced and different political affiliations seem to neutralize the effect of such remote kinship. (Ibid.: 24)

The only other implication of these disparate clan memberships is that one may not eat all or part of one's taboo animal. The bans are still strongly observed in my experience. I was surprised and puzzled, early in my work in Mutare, to come upon a headline in the local newspaper, the *Manica Post* (a government-owned paper with a decidedly tabloid editorial policy), that read: 'Crowd beats up meat vendor'. Intrigued, I read further. The crowd in question had heard via rumour or some other more authenticated source that a particular seller of meat in a market was, in fact, selling monkey meat under the guise of something else. The reaction only makes sense in terms of an understanding that many people in the market belonged to the clan *shoko* and were in danger of being duped into eating their clan animal by an unscrupulous dealer. (The danger of eating your totem animal is that 'your teeth will fall out or you will otherwise become ill,' most people say when asked).

A reading of the anthropological literature on 'the Shona' is an experience in watching the material change before one's eyes. The earliest writers (Charles Bullock, 1928, for example) name only groups such as the Karanga, the Korekore, or the Zezuru, for example and not the conglomeration now referred to as Shona. The focus in their writings is on specificity confined by geography, locale or local authority (in particular, specific chiefdoms). And we have seen, in the previous chapter, frank admissions from major anthropologists that the umbrella term 'Shona' was itself a construct of colonial rule. It is interesting to see that, already in 1952, Holleman is noting the gradual change in 'custom', here read sorrowfully as 'a rule breaking down'. The attention to change and the impact of urbanization and 'culture contact' were all, of course, central to the research concerns of Gluckman and the work of the Rhodes-Livingstone Institute (again, see Werbner 1984 and Schumaker 2001).

The anthropological subject has always been a moving object, as Edmund Leach, an important figure in British social anthropology, pointed out:

> Social anthropology is packed with frustrations of this kind. An obvious example is the category opposition patrilineal/matrilineal. Ever since Morgan began writing of the Iroquois, it has been customary for anthropologists to distinguish unilineal from non-unilineal

descent systems, and among the former to distinguish patrilineal societies from matrilineal societies. These categories now seem to us so rudimentary and obvious that it is extremely difficult to break out of the straitjacket of thought which the categories themselves impose. (Leach 1961: 3)

In this passage, from his famous critique of comparative methods in the anthropological study of kinship systems, Leach challenges the very foundations of classificatory binaries in ideas of culturally variant approaches to family and relatedness. Indeed, I believe it could be argued that the far-ranging deconstruction of anthropological accounts of kinship (a matter that dominated late 20th century anthropology) began, at this moment, with Leach. He goes further:

It is some years since Professor Firth drew attention to the alarming proliferation of structuralist terminology .... That was in 1951, but the process has continued. We now have not merely filiation but complementary filiation, not merely siblings but residual siblings. Of such cycles and epicycles there is no end. (Ibid.: 26)

Holleman, working in the 1940s (and writing in 1952), is describing the Hera peoples of central Shona country, and deliberately seeking out those 'less contaminated by change' (now often referred to as the 'deep rural'). Describing Shona kinship from the perspective of a growing boy (a perspective Michael Gelfand employed in 1979), Holleman gives a description of the emerging, widening realm of kinship and links it directly to residential locality (that is, you come to know 'family' as those with whom you live from a young age):

Growing up he [his putative boy] recognizes the individual members of his family as representatives of specific types of relations which recur again and again as he gets acquainted with a widening circle of kindred. Amongst his agnates the graded scale of seniority and rank is extended beyond the children of his own father, amongst his collaterals in other branches of his lineage. His own father assumes a position in a likewise graded succession of 'fathers'. At family rituals (*bira*) he perceives that this hierarchy of the living links up with the world of the dead, whose spirits, too, have their individual places in the agnatic order. The structure of his patrilineage is unfolded as a growing entity split into different but component parts of various sizes. His own family is but one of numerous similar units which link up in more-enveloping units. But the connections between these units are individuals who, like himself, occupy a fixed position as relatively senior or junior, superior or subordinate, in an ever-extending order of succession. (Holleman 1952: 60)

This is a clear example of the form of highly technical, functionalist versions of kinship theory that Leach so presciently critiqued. However, for the moment, let us continue along this tightrope of accounts of kinship, while trying to remain aware that the subjects (the 'Shona') and the structures ('patrilineal kinship') are all, to some extent, constructed under specific and highly problematic conditions of colonial classification and domination. For example, Benedict Anderson (1983) has meticulously documented how, for colonialism and nationalism, the census and the map, the classification of space and types of people were central to the colonial project. Let us also take note of the fact that Holleman already acknowledges change as a feature of the systems he describes, albeit in the language of nostalgia and lament.

Kinship in a time of war

The next major ethnography of the Shona was the work of Michael Bourdillon. He is an anthropologist and former Jesuit priest, trained at Oxford under E.E. Evans-Pritchard. Bourdillon conducted the bulk of his fieldwork in north-eastern Zimbabwe in the late 1960s, amongst the Korekore sub-group, prior to the intense civil war known as the Second Chimurenga (see Mtsi, Nyakudya and Barnes, 2009, for an historical account of the period and the elements of valorization in its written history. Chimurenga translates as 'uprising'). He was particularly interested in the religious beliefs and practices of the Shona set squarely in the context of pervasive social change, explicitly including urbanization and cash economies.

This may be an appropriate moment to consider the very important role of missionaries in the development of the ethnography of the Shona peoples. Herbert Plangger, Herbert Aschwanden (1989), Hubert Bucher (1980) and Marthinus Daneel (1971) were all Christian missionaries who contributed substantially to the development of Shona ethnographies (especially, as did Bourdillon, to explications of Shona cosmologies). Peter Pels, in his review of the anthropology of colonialism, remarks:

> Urged by the necessity to communicate the Gospel, missionaries did probably more substantial recording of unknown languages than all anthropologists taken together. Because learning a language implies learning cultural competence, they also had to cope with the relations of power that are constructed by and expressed in hierarchies between languages, their notation and translation, and the conversations that occurred on that basis .... Thus, the combination of religious teaching, massive involvement in colonial education, and relative autonomy from the practice of colonial control gave missionaries a special position at the juncture of colonial technologies of domination and self-control. (Pels 1997: 171-2)

Bourdillon's major work, *The Shona Peoples* (1976) was published at the height of the civil war but was based on material collected in the 1960s and from secondary sources. As he has noted, fieldwork was impossible during the years of violence (roughly 1968 to 1980)[1]. Bourdillon is explicit about the constraints and limitations of doing fieldwork and writing ethnography in times of immense social change as colonial domination came to an end. Yet, like Holleman,

---

[1] Michael Bourdillon, 2010, personal communication. In the next section I rely heavily on Bourdillon's accounts of Shona kinship. Long quotations are clumsy so I have adopted the strategy of putting the central part of the quote in the text while the rest may be found in the accompanying footnote, for those interested in greater detail.

he is primarily concerned with rural livelihoods and lives, although he is also concerned to relate his descriptions of rural practice to urban experiences and changes (although not to resurgent African nationalism). I mention this to stress that the cultural groupings here referred to as the Shona peoples are fluid, dynamic and changing. This is as true of their ideas and practices of kinship as it is of other aspects of their cultural formations. However, the following description of Shona patrilineal practice and language will be instructive in my ethnography to follow:

> In their use of kinship terms people distinguish members of their own patrilineal group only by generation, age and sex, and not according to genealogical distance.[2] (Bourdillon 1976: 26)

Bourdillon notes in his analysis that these forms of the patrilineal were reinforced by common residential patterns of rural/pre-urban Shona society.[3]

[2] 'Thus the term *baba* (father) can mean a father's brother or any man in the patriclan belonging to the father's generation: a distinction may be made between *baba mukuru* (great father), who is senior to one's father, and *baba mudiki* (little father), who is junior, but there is no titular distinction between, for example, father's brother and father's distant cousin (provided they are all in the same clan). Similarly all females in the father's generation and belonging to the same clan are called *vatete* (paternal aunt) no matter how distantly they are related. A man calls the men of his generation *mukoma* or *munun'una* depending on whether they are older or younger than himself, and the same terms are used by women of women. The term *mwana* (sometimes specified as *mwanakomana* for a boy and *mwanasikana* for a girl) applies equally to a child and to any other clan member of one's children's generation.' Bourdillon 1976: 26.

[3] 'It used to be, and often still is, the ambition of a man to gather around him a growing lineage of descendants and dependants, who would act as a corporate body for economic purposes and also as a united body in times of crisis or tension in the community. And so the sons of a family grew up in an extended (rather than an elementary) family that included their paternal grandparents, their parents, their father's brothers and their wives, their brother and sisters and their patrilineal cousins .... Although the extended kinship terminology has always applied to a wider group of people, close family ties were normally recognized in practice *only between those who lived together*.' Ibid.: 27. My emphasis.

I want to call this a preferred version of Shona kinship, amongst Shona people themselves as much as among anthropologists. And I pointedly emphasize the exception that comes here at the end of Bourdillon's paean to 'what used to be'. (Nostalgia and idealization are never very far behind in kinship theory, I would venture to suggest). For, in fact, Bourdillon (and even the more conservative Holleman) recount numerous exceptions to general rules. Here is one significant exception, from Bourdillon, to the 'rule' of patrilineal, virilocal residence:

> Even prior to modern influences there were variations in residence patterns. A poor man, for example, who was not able to pay bride-price cattle could instead spend his life working for his father-in-law: in such a situation he would leave his own extended family and join his wife's.[4] (Ibid.: 28)

I emphasize the exception here as a way to counter the prevailing force of 'ideal patrilineal family structure' in much writing, and talking, about Shona families and kin systems. There were certainly always dominant patterns and preferred forms, but they were by no means universal and a wide variety of alternatives have been found. As Bourdillon notes in the section above, one primary outlet for the expression and performance of alternatives was the wife's/mother's family. The powerful role of the mother, and her kin (in particular her brother), needs to be remarked upon, even in relation to

---

[4] 'In some areas (in the Zambezi valley, for example, where the tsetse fly curbed herds of cattle) it was normal procedure for a man to live and work for his wife's father until his own daughters were married; then he was likely to build his own independent homestead rather than return to his father's home. In this area homesteads were always smaller than in central Shona country where they could grow into nuclear village communities. *Apart from these institutionalized variations, it is always possible for a man to live with friends, in-laws or close kin who are not of his patrilineage, whether because of conflict with his own family or because of a particularly close relationship with his new neighbours. In practice not all residential groups conform to the ideal family structure*'. (Ibid.: 28. My emphasis)

idealized versions of Shona kinship:

> At the death of a mother, her spirit is regarded as friendly and pro-
> tective. Some say that maternal spirit elders are more important than
> spirits of patrilineal ancestors and that nothing harmful can happen
> to a person without the consent of his maternal spirits.[5] (Ibid.: 32)

Nor are these close and spiritually powerful relationships with one's
mother confined to the afterlife either:

> The relationship of a Shona person towards his or her mother's line-
> age is quite different from that between members of the same line-
> age. The women of the mother's lineage are all called *mai* (mother)
> and the relationship with these women is typified by the mother-
> child relationship: *one of these women may well replace the mother should
> she die young.*[6] (Ibid.: 33. My emphasis)

We might then say that relationships with one's mother and with
her family are relationships marked by especially strong affective
bonds, as well as cross-generational intimacies not normally seen in

---

[5] 'This is reflected in the exclamation, *"Maiwe!"* [my mother!], so commonly
uttered in distress: it is the spirit of the mother who is supposed to have caused
the trouble or at least to have allowed it. Because the mother carried the off-
spring in her womb, underwent pregnancy and the pains of labour, and nour-
ished and cared for them while they were helpless children, at the death of the
mother her spirit demands to be well remembered and honoured .... Maternal
spirit elders are so important as custodians of a child's well-being that occasionally a child's father's family waives its legal rights over a sick child in order
to allow it to live with its maternal kin who can more readily communicate with
its maternal spirits.' (Ibid.: 32)

[6] 'The relationship with men of the mother's lineage is typified in the relationship between a mother's brother and his sister's son, a relationship which
plays a prominent role in many ritual and social situations. This relationship is
expressed in the complementary terms *sekuru* (mother's brother) and *muzukuru*
(sister's son) – the uses of these terms are of course extended to include other
members of the lineages concerned .... Even unrelated persons can adopt the
terms *sekuru* and *muzukuru* towards each other to express a friendly relationship, reflecting the typical relationship between mother's brother and sister's
son." (Ibid.: 33)

the patriclan with the exception of the grandparent/grandchild relationship, which on both father's and mother's side is a site of love, unreserved, and (as we shall see) instantiated in profound ways. In his account of Shona childhoods, Michael Gelfand (1979) notes that children were routinely sent to stay with either set of grandparents after they had been weaned from the breast (about two years old). This was the case, in his study, whether either children or grandparents were living in rural or urban areas. His informants told him that the primary reason for this practice (which is mentioned in older ethnographies as well) was that grandparents were very 'loving' to their grandchildren, and were good at teaching children 'manners'. In addition small children were said to be useful for small errands.

From function and structure to practice in kinship theory

I have mined the older ethnographic literature for both its descriptions of an idealized structure of relatedness and for hints of variations from ideal norms of family practice. I do this in order to bolster my own ethnographic findings where I was often surprised to find that children, with a few exceptions, were being (and had been) cared for by their mothers or their mother's relatives.

However, first we must consider both the radical change brought about in Zimbabwe with the end of colonialism in 1980,[7] and anthropology's disenchantment with both functionalist and structuralist accounts of kinship. The latter, of course, was a process that had begun prior even to Bourdillon's last bold attempt at a grand nar-

---

[7]   See James Muzondidya (2009) and Brian Raftopoulos (2009) for accounts of the historical circumstances constituting the post-colonial period in Zimbabwe. Historians have been particularly active in developing rigorous academic accounts of both the far and recent past in the construction of contemporary Zimbabwe. Terence Ranger (1985) is pre-eminent. See also Ranger, McGregor and Alexander (2000) and Alexander (2006). For pre-colonial Zimbabwean history see the works of David Beech (for example, 1980).

rative of Shona culture(s). I have here suggested that the shift in anthropology's theorizing of kinship began in 1961 with Edmund Leach's Malinowski Lecture as quoted above. I do not intend to give an account of the complex evolution of kinship studies within anthropology. Such accounts are lengthy and have been undertaken to great effect elsewhere (for example, Schneider 1968, Peletz 1995, Collier and Yanagisako 1987, Carston 2004). In his review, Michael Peletz summarizes the preoccupations of late 20th century kinship studies:

> Contemporary kinship studies tend to be historically grounded; tend to focus on everyday experiences, understandings, and representations of gender, power and difference; and tend to devote considerable analytic attention to themes of contradiction, paradox and ambivalence. (Peletz 1995: 367)

Nor is this a place for a summary of Zimbabwe's complex, and frequently tragic post-colonial history. Brian Raftoupoulos and Alois Mlambo (2009) have just published a remarkably comprehensive overview of the period, and further analysis has become available in the past decade of 'crisis'.[8]

However, I shall comment on two studies that emerged in post-colonial Zimbabwe that have a bearing on our subject here. The first was the acclaimed publication, in 1981, of David Lan's *Guns and Rain: Guerillas and Spirit Mediums in Zimbabwe*. Lan's ethnography was an account of the relationships developed during the long years of the bush guerilla war, in the remote north-eastern Dande area, between guerillas (as the harbingers of the new, particularly of forms of Maoist/socialist rhetoric and practice) and senior spirit mediums (as guardians of the land and the rain, and as conduits between the

---

[8] In a rapidly growing body of work see for example, Hammar, Raftoupoulos and Jensen (2003), Harold-Barry (2004), Raftoupolos and Savage (2005) Hammar, McGregor and Landau (2010). These are all edited collections. From anthropology see Moore (2005) and Bornstein (2005).

living and the dead). In his dramatic account the *vakomana* (boys: the common vernacular term for the guerillas who were often young men or adolescents) are idealized as the principled defenders of common people against the brutal colonial/settler forces, and are guided in their struggle by the powers of the ancestral spirits through the direct intervention of the spirit mediums. Besides the *vakomana*, the involvement of children and young people was considerably broadened by the activities of *mujibhas* (young boys) and *chimbwidos* (young girls) who undertook tasks such as carrying supplies, scouting, spying and carrying messages. Their role and its risk should not be underplayed.

The work reads as a gripping account of popular resistance through hybrids of the modern and the autochthonous. A cursory reading of the reviews it received from fellow scholars at the time of its publication shows how rapturously it was received by most, although there were exceptions, most notably Bourdillon, who questioned its fieldwork base and its highly simplistic account of Shona spirit mediums (and their notoriously internecine quarrels).

The fate of the work, acclaimed at publication as the very model of a new form of ethnography (and anthropology) that could re-invigorate a discipline heavily tainted by its colonial connections, has uncannily mirrored the post-colonial state it sought so vividly and positively to represent in its first promising moment. Both (ex-) guerillas and spirit mediums have suffered severely in the popular imagination as a result of their various attachments to the ruling party (see Mtisi, Nyakudya and Barnes 2009, Kriger 2003), and perhaps their lack of attachment to popular Christianity (Maxwell 2006). The extensive historical work of Terence Ranger and others has developed a more nuanced and compelling account of the liberation war and its aftermath (see Ranger 1985, for a work that came out in the same period, dealing with the natures and forms of the liberation war, but that has weathered significantly better).

The other major anthropological contribution of the first decades of post-colonial Zimbabwe was the work of Pamela Reynolds (1991, 1996). Reynolds' work is particularly instructive as it was the first serious, sustained attempt to examine the lives of children in Zimbabwe through an ethnographic lens. In *Dance Civet Cat: Child Labour in the Zambezi Valley* (1991), she meticulously examined the labour of children within agrarian households amongst Tonga people (a non-Shona, matrilineal grouping). In the course of the work she demonstrated that children were able to develop considerable degrees of autonomy through the strategic offering of their labour, and through it, to develop some kin ties in preference to others. She was also able to show that children were responsible for a significant portion of labour in marginal, drought-prone subsistence economies. She concluded:

> We can learn something of value about childhood if we carefully examine children's recognition and use of the options society offers in defining the rules of kinship. I am suggesting that children partly negotiate their own fate .... Support is not given equally to all who fall within the category sanctioned by kin norms. The relationship is negotiated: the child's role is an active one. (Reynolds 1991: 143-4)

In her next work, *Traditional Healers and Childhood in Zimbabwe*, (1996), Reynolds examined the relationship between children and traditional healers (in this case primarily among the Zezuru, another Shona sub-group, people living around Musami in the north-east), and once again would demonstrate through meticulous observation that children were active labourers alongside their elders in the healing enterprise, had extensive knowledge of local pharmacopeia and were active agents in developing and maintaining preferred kinship ties. Reynolds' work sits interestingly alongside that of Lan. If both had an interest in the young and their relationship with forms of the old (traditional healers and kinship structure respectively), they are marked as far apart in other respects. Reynolds's fieldwork is rigorous and detailed, her subjects more precisely situated.

Reynolds' work allows us a way back into more contemporary perspectives on kinship and family in Zimbabwe. In many ways her portrayal of children and their families comes close to what John Borneman has referred to as the central process in defining relatedness; 'the process of caring and being cared for' (2001: 31). The idea of 'process' is essential here: a sustained living out of the possibilities of relatedness through the performance of daily acts of mutual care. It is within this framework that I wish now to turn to my own ethnographic material from eastern Zimbabwe, as described in the previous chapter.

From my own ethnography of a wide range of material I select a few cases that will exemplify both the continuing hold of older forms and beliefs in a metastructure of patrilineal kinship, and a daily practice of care under circumstances of dire extremity in which variations within the metastructure are common.

Struggle and grief in families: a case study

Let us consider the experience of one young girl whom I have called Priscilla. She was fourteen when I met her five years ago, although to me she looked no more than ten or eleven on first sight. She is still (some years later now) short and thin, almost skeletally so. Her hair is sparse; the skin on her face and arms is mottled with a rash. Priscilla is obviously not healthy. She has a tense and animated air, and an articulateness that immediately belies her appearance. Like the other children in the group she slips in speech between English and Shona, but she is verbally skilled, articulate, eager and able to speak up for the others and on her own behalf. A leader, then, not least because she is the first to identify herself as being HIV-positive, when others murmur of TB or some vague sickness. I see a child eager to engage, competent in relating to others, charming, and resilient.

Priscilla is an orphan, a double orphan in the language of public health in which she is referred to me by local health professionals, meaning that both her parents are dead. Her father died when she was an infant and she has no memories of him although she knows that her parents were estranged and in dispute over maintenance payments. Her mother died when she was about nine. She had lived with her mother and her maternal grandmother, and when her mother died she continued to live with her grandmother, with whom she was very close and who seems to have played a crucial role in mediating the loss of her mother. 'She took me to the funeral even when others said I was too young, and she even showed me the body when no one was looking. She was very loving to me. She bought me these shoes. They are the last new shoes I ever had.'

Priscilla has mixed memories of her mother who, for as long as she can remember, was very ill. Her illness made her remote and unavailable, and also, guiltily, burdensome. 'But sometimes she was better and she would hold me, and laugh, and be loving.' By contrast her grandmother was lively, nurturing, and care-giving. She died of cancer when Priscilla was eleven and it is this loss that lingers for her, overwhelming and evoking the other losses, and marking a new kind of aloneness.

It is a loss that is still fresh, bringing tears to her eyes. 'They would not let me see her in the hospital as they said she was too sick and I was too young but one of the nurses told me that, when she died, she was calling for me.' Priscilla speaks of her dreams of both her mother and grandmother: 'they smile at me, my mother smiles, and my grandmother tells me to be good and laughs.' This is comforting, but she identifies 'home' as being where they are. When she feels most dislocated and alone, it is the sense of loved ones waiting for her in a spirit world that she is homesick for. 'I think heaven is a very peaceful place to be. I hope I can go there.'

Priscilla is the middle child of three girls. Her elder sister, Patricia, was eighteen when I first met Priscilla and living with a man in Harare with whom she had a young child. Patricia had told Priscilla that she was going to get married in order to be able to provide a home for her young sisters. Unfortunately her relationship with her partner is very difficult and marked by domestic violence. The promised reunion of the sisters in her home has not materialized, and Priscilla has only seen her twice since moving to Mutare three years ago. Her younger sister, Charity, is nine. At the time of their grandmother's death, a family conference was held in which it was decided by the adult members of her maternal family that Priscilla should go to live with her maternal aunt in Mutare while Charity should go to her maternal grandfather in Bulawayo (the two cities are some 800km distant from each other). The separation of the two younger sisters marks the other great loss of Priscilla's life. She speaks often of her, has little contact with her and fears for her health. Her sister is also HIV-positive.

The home of her maternal aunt, Mrs Gwaunza, is a crowded one. It consists of four small rooms. Besides her aunt and uncle and their three children, there is a nephew of her aunt's husband and (like Priscilla) an orphan. Both adults are employed: her aunt manages a minibus that her cousin drives and her uncle is a low-ranking civil servant. There is little money to spare and many competing demands for its use, and (perhaps inevitably) that gives Priscilla's descriptions a constant undertone of the fair and the unfair. She is articulate about the minutiae of daily slights, sorrows and minor graces. One day she described for me the pain, neglect and anger she felt when, at a family meal, all the children were served with chicken drumsticks, while she was given a wing. Another time, having neglected to make her bed in the rush to get to school, she came home to find her blankets had been soaked 'as punishment' and she was beaten by her aunt for this. These were punishments that seem to me to be out of proportion to the offences, and to Priscilla they rankled as deeply unfair, although much of her interaction within the family seems to elicit a similar rage against injustice, enhanced by comparison with her remembered, idealized, and lost position of love and care in her grandmother's household.

In a crowded house with few resources, much must be shared, and adults must make frequent, hard decisions about the allocation of resources, mediating as best they can amongst competing demands. For the children the demands include bedding, food, clothing and access to money from the household budget. Priscilla is acutely aware of the hard choices and yet considers herself to be a low priority for her aunt and uncle, because of her more distant kinship status. (Priscilla is, formally, distant kin as she lives with maternal kin in a patrilineal society where, as the common saying goes, 'your mother's relatives are strangers'). Her elder cousin, for example, goes to a boarding school and she sees this as a privilege since the one boarding is spared the shortages of food and the demands of daily chores that must be borne by those at home. For many children I know, boarding school is seen as a privilege since it allows uninterrupted study, more regular food (in quantity if not quality) and opportunities for the development of close friendships.

One day I visited the Gwaunza household, and was received with honour in an immaculate though crowded front living room. On one side hung two inscriptions: 'Lord', invoked the first, 'allow my enemies to live a long life so that they may see my progress. Amen', while the other was both more pointed and more terse (at least for the ethnographer and certainly for any Zimbabwean attuned to the constant fear of state surveillance): 'Be a true visitor, not a spy.' Suitably admonished, I was entertained by Priscilla's aunt and uncle who were keen to hear my sense of her wellbeing. They both said that they thought she was doing well within the household, seemed more self-confident, and was doing reasonably well at school. But the larger issue raised for me was one I had often heard alluded to by Priscilla, which was that of secrecy, and bad luck. 'Yes', they said to me, 'she has had a hard time, very bad luck. And it keeps happening. The bad luck seems to follow her.' They acknowledged hesitantly that they had consulted a *n'anga* about whether there might be an *ngozi* (an aggrieved ancestral spirit) responsible for the 'bad luck'. He had been non-committal, but they remained disconcerted. These were serious matters if the occult was implicated. It seemed to me that it was but a short step from having bad luck to being bad luck, and beyond that lay the spectres of aggrieved spirits and even witchcraft. This is the reported version of the outcome of their consultation. I think it unlikely that a healer would have been 'non-committal' and I wonder whether this conversation indicated Priscilla's aunt and uncle as having some guilt about their treatment of her. Guilt at the treatment of a child would also give rise to fear of ancestral anger, as children are especially dear to family spirits.

Priscilla felt that her life was constantly marked by a sense of secrecy. Her aunt and uncle told her that she should be circumspect in her descriptions of herself and where she lived. 'Just say that your parents are working outside of the country,' she reported to me that they said to her. And, indeed, this would be an unremarkable commonplace in everyday Zimbabwe. Another time she told me of being teased by other children at school: 'You are so thin and small, you must have AIDS,' they said. She was rescued by a fellow group member to whom she has become close, but experienced a moment of sharp panic when she felt as though she had nothing to say in her own defence.

Priscilla's willingness to admit to being HIV-positive is restricted to the group. Like many of the children she is very unwilling to discuss her health in other social settings. For example, at church she tells me she 'prays in her heart' about her fears and tribulations, of antiretrovirals and marked illnesses but would not dream of eliciting the attention and support of her fellow worshippers, at least some of whom must be in a similar situation.

I have chosen Priscilla's story here as one that exemplifies many of the themes that have emerged as I have come to know children and their carers, and that is the dominant role that maternal kin play in the care of orphaned children. Priscilla does know who her paternal kin are and where they are. As we have seen, her parents were formally married even though the marriage ended and her parents were involved in divorce proceedings at the time of her father's death. Her father is dead and she has heard that two of his brothers are also dead. She has met one paternal uncle (*baba munini*/small father) when he visited her aunt's house some years ago, and she believes that this visit was primarily to check on her welfare as this is what her aunt told her at the time. She knows that her paternal grandmother lives in a rural community near Murewa in the northeast of Zimbabwe (borderline Zezuru/Korekore country). She has heard too that her grandmother is a traditional healer, with knowledge of healing herbs, and she claims that this makes her fearful of meeting this grandmother 'because she might be a witch'. She knows of no attempts that her paternal grandmother has initiated in order to see her. She imagines that she will have no contact with her paternal kin until she needs them. This 'need' is foreseen as the time when she marries, and formal marriage negotiations will require the involvement of her paternal kin.

The forms and sorrows of marriage: a case study

This is an appropriate time for a description of Shona conceptions of marriage which, if one may summarize, is perceived as a lengthy process rather than a single event, and as a contract between families (lineages) rather than between individuals. While noting that much has changed and that many variations occur, Bourdillon usefully describes the processes of Shona marriage thus:

> I have argued that marriage among the Shona is primarily a contract between groups rather than between individuals. Another way in which Shona marriage is a drawn-out process: there is no clear point at which the couple can say that they are now married whereas they were not married before. To explain this we must look at the normal marriage procedures and payments, that is, in the sense that they are

considered the correct ideal, not in the sense that they are always or even usually followed.[9] (Bourdillon op.cit: 41)

It should be noted that even this elaborate process was not considered conclusive. One might even say that it is debatable that Shona marriage was ever considered entirely complete. Firstly, it might take the lifetime of the groom to complete payments, which were never expected all at once. The state of ongoing indebtedness to the wife's family allowed the latter to be able to call on their *mukwasha* (son-in-law) for help and labour at critical moments. Secondly, sterility, adultery or any form of abuse would severely affect or even reverse the process. In particular a woman's failure to get pregnant was a grave impediment to further solidifying the marriage and often seen as grounds for divorce or at least a sign that it would be wise for the man to take a second (hopefully more fruitful) wife. Thirdly, the option of the man taking other wives remains a common and viable one. The 'traditional' version of polygamy would be that a man would take second or third wives when he became wealthy enough (since all had to have their own homesteads and cooking huts), effectively

[9] 'Informal courting moves into a private engagement by the exchange of love tokens between the boy and girl, often passed through a third person ... Although sexual intercourse is not strictly allowed at this stage and the girl should certainly not be made pregnant, the exchange of love tokens is often a prelude to sexual intercourse and nowadays does not always indicate intention to marry .... The engagement becomes more formal and public when the suitor approaches the girl's family. The first approaches are made through an intermediary or "messenger" who is related to neither family and who is an important witness should a subsequent dispute arise ... who enters the homestead and explains the nature of his visit to a responsible person, handing him a token gift. This is usually passed on to the girl's father, who indicates his agreement by accepting the gift .... From this point on the reciprocal terms *mukwasha* (son-in-law) and *tezvara* (father-in-law) are adopted indicating that the affinal relationship has been established ... [Further negotiations through the messenger ensue] It has always involved two payments ... *rustambo* (the first payment) is associated with sexual rights to the woman ... *roora* (the second payment) is associated with rights over children born to the woman.' (Ibid.: 41)

restricting the practice to a few. My own observation is that 'modern' polygamy involves a less overtly practiced form, where wives live in separate areas and common language refers to *mai guru* (senior wife) and *mai'nini* (junior wife), *imba mukuru*/big houses and *imba mudiki*/small houses (junior wives, of course, being the occupants of smaller houses) or even the English term 'mistresses'. Finally, couples and their families who belong to Christian churches, now a majority, insert a church wedding (and a civil legal contract) into this process. My observation is that such a ceremony often happens after the birth of at least one child. Marriage without children seems particularly meaningless to many Shona people I know. Indeed it should be borne in mind that true adulthood was not traditionally thought to have been achieved until one had become a parent. The childless adult is an anomalous and potentially dangerous figure in these forms of Shona cosmology. I should know, for I occupy this eerie place myself.

Takura was a 16-year-old boy who lived with his mother and his 14-year-old brother when I met them four years ago. All three are HIV-positive. Takura's father is dead. He died of an AIDS-related illness some five years ago. He was a very successful man who had begun as the driver in a major international NGO working in reproductive health and HIV infection in Manicaland, and from this relatively lowly position, he had risen in the organization to become a community development officer. He came from a Manyika family and had met his future wife, a Karanga woman who at that time was living with her family near Masvingo (some 300km south-west), in the course of his travels for work. He had courted her in the traditional ways and some three years after meeting she had moved to Mutare to set up house with him. The various bride-price payments had been, or were in the process of being, paid. After the birth of their second son, the couple also had a wedding in the Roman Catholic Church. At this time, they had their own house in the high-density suburb of Dangamvura. Takura's father fell ill. Takura's mother told me that, by this time, she suspected that he had another woman but that they did not discuss this as she felt she had no grounds for complaint as she was well cared for.

When Takura's father fell ill, his family (his mother and his elder brother) arrived after some weeks and took him, together with his family, to see a renowned *n'anga* in the Chipinge area. The *n'anga* announced that the ill man had been possessed by a healing *shave* (an alien spirit) and that he was being called to be a healer (we shall explore these ideas about different forms of spirits in later chapters). Takura's father continued to worsen and, a few months later, he died. His family arrived at the widow's house and reclaimed all his possessions. Without any means of support, she was forced to live with her brother and sister-in-law. She tells me that her late husband's family did not offer to assist her and that her mother-in-law even accused her of having bewitched her late son. Takura's mother was especially upset by this accusation since she had hoped that the earlier involvement of the *n'anga* would have spared her this accusation. He had explicitly not attributed the late man's sickness to witchcraft. Inheritance and the fate of widows in the face of greedy relatives of their late husband's has been the subject of much debate[10] in Zimbabwe over the past two decades. Consider the following:

> In the traditional inheritance systems, widows do not receive any of the deceased's property, though they do keep their own personal effects including any personal gifts the husband may have made over to them during his life. In the rural subsistence economy, a widow continues to work the fields her late husband allocated to her and she is cared for either by his relatives or by her own family if she refuses to accept an inheritor. In the urban situation, however, a widow

[10] By debate I refer to frequent local press coverage of such cases where widows are reduced to poverty following the deaths of their husbands and the actions of their husbands' relatives. For examples see the archives at www.misa.co.zw. The matter is rightly seen by the UN as a clear contravention of gender equality and women's rights (see www.unhcr.org).

may well be left destitute by her husband's kin who often claim all his property, including house furniture and items purchased with the husband's and wife's joint income, immediately on the death of their kinsman and without bothering to decide who is responsible for the maintenance of the widow. The traditional rules of inheritance applied outside the context of the extended family structure and without the traditional social restraints can have disastrous social consequences. (Ibid.: 216)

When I met the family (or its bereaved remnants) some three years later, Mai Takura was subsisting largely on her brother's charity, although in recent years he too had begun to sicken and she feared greatly for the future. She supplemented the family's income with sporadic market work, selling vegetables and home-baked scones. Both of these money-making ventures had been severely disrupted by military action against, first, the urban poor and their street markets, and secondly, by the ruthless crushing of the diamond trade.[11] She had had herself and her sons tested for HIV about six months after the death of her husband and they had all tested positive. It is the belief of both doctors and their mother that the boys have been HIV-positive since birth. She described herself to me as 'a graduate of HIV'. Her grief was palpable and fresh, made more onerous by what she perceived as her having been abandoned by her husband's family. 'Who was the witch?' she asked me bitterly. Mostly, her thoughts were preoccupied with her sons, now teenagers, who had only faint memories of their father. Takura was the frailer of the two. He had frequent chest infections and bouts of diarrhoea. He looked younger than his younger brother, and this rankled. The two boys quarreled for a variety of reasons.

In one thing, though, Mai Takura's sons were united. They were devoted to her, and anxious for her wellbeing. 'If I get sick, they

[11] See footnote 12, p.29, for references relevant to Operation Murambatsvina and, in Mutare, its interpellation with the ongoing Chiadzwa diamond debacle.

do everything for me,' she said with a quiet pride, 'and if I am late home they will come looking for me.' This reduced family unit, Mai Takura, her brother, her sister-in-law, and their five children had become a small, self-caring, resilient group that did not look for or expect to find help outside of their small circle. When I asked Takura and his brother about their paternal relatives, I was curtly told 'they are dead' (*vakafa*). Their mother tells me that she does not think that this is true; she has heard that other members of her husband's family are alive, but she has not seen them and has heard only vague rumours. She tells me that she would like her sons to have contact with their father's family, 'but it is not my place to seek that'. She believes them to be in need of the 'protection' of their father's family although when I ask her explicitly if she means the care of paternal elder spirits, she changes the subject.

Depleted and fictional kin

Thinking about the disparate experiences of Priscilla and Takura who have both found care in their mother's families, I am puzzled again by this most common of Shona sayings, *'your mother's relatives are strangers'*.[12] For on the most concrete and practical of levels it is clearly not true. I would in fact venture the opposite opinion. In dire need, it is your mother's family who are most likely to care for you. In the case of Priscilla (and many other children I know) what is immediately striking is that, in the absence of a parent or grandparent, the frequent outcome for children is one of displacement through a variety of households within their mother's side of the family, through which parenting is provided by a wide variety of adult kin, including aunts, uncles, elder siblings and other affines.

One of the chief limitations of this otherwise elastic approach to the provision of care hinges, it seems to me, on the separation of siblings. Being separated from her sisters is the single greatest factor

---

[12] See Hamutyinei and Plangger, (1974).

driving Priscilla's sense of isolation, although here again we may be wise to consider the roles of nostalgia and idealization even as they work in the most intimate recesses of domesticity. For, by way of sharp contrast, Takura and his brother are antagonistic in everything but their concern for their mother. Perhaps fights between siblings are another form of intimacy, preferable to separation, especially the extreme, long-distance separation experienced by Priscilla and her sisters.

In the cases I have cited, the other startling fact, partly concealed by layers of internecine fighting, is the severe depletion of the number of kin available. The harsh fact is that there are simply not many people left in families. Persistence lived with his mother, his younger brother, his mother's youngest sister and her three children. Persistence knew of only two members of his father's family who were still alive and they were two of his father's sisters, his *vatete*. His father, his paternal grandparents and his paternal uncles are all dead. This is a domestic, familial landscape of wholesale death, of absence and of cumulative bereavement.

One way in which this depletion and loss is staunched is through the development and maintenance of fictive kin. I have already alluded to the ways in which I have been, over time and with some initial hesitance, adopted as *sekuru* (mother's brother), *baba* (father, or father's brother) and *mukoma* (brother). Anyone, however, who has been in Zimbabwe, for even a short time, will have experienced something similar. It is simply deemed polite to give strangers, especially adults, kin titles. (My own enthusiastic attempts to encourage everyone to call me by my first name, a sign of friendliness within another cultural domain, have never been successful). However I find it fruitful to think about it in terms of an invitation to enter a relationship of intimacy, defined by the potentials and constraints of parallel kin relationships.

Isaiah, a 19-year-old who I have known for some years, scrupulously refers to me as his father. In the context of our relationship I

79

understand this to be an invitation to help care for him more, to help alleviate his unending struggle against dire poverty. It is, however, also a sign of his willingness to perform the role of my child: to do things for me, to listen to my advice and to accept my admonitions. He lives with his elderly paternal grandmother who also refers to me, repeatedly and with emphasis, as *baba waIsaiah* (the father of Isaiah). Isaiah's real father has been dead for more than ten years and his mother for more than twelve. His grandmother raised him, and his two older brothers, with some small help from her daughter, who is widowed and who has three children of her own to care for.

I have seen similar patterns elsewhere. Aunty Thandi, who runs the church office, is everyone's *tete* (father's sister). She is routinely called this by children and carers alike. And she performs the role of slightly stern, although affectionate, moral guardian with aplomb. A domain in which I have never seen the offering or receiving of terms of fictive kinship is the hospital, where all staff are very submissively referred to by professional titles, *masister* (nurse) and *chiremba* (doctor). Schools and churches offer another example of the same highly formalized patterns of interaction. Teachers and pastors are always referred to with honorific titles (*mufundisi*/teacher). This is interesting. It is not a matter of brief relationships. All of the children I know well have seen the same doctors and nurses since birth. They often see them every three months (considerably more often than they see many of their own close kin), and yet the spoken performance of the relationship remains highly formalized.

Spiritual families

Perhaps the ultimate form of fictive kin is to be found in the realm of the spiritual. God is the ultimate father, and it is Jesus who cares most. The everyday forms of caring performed in homes and neighbourhoods are understood by my informants as essential, but also as pale reflections, and frail earthly instantiations, of the intense love and care of God. Ideals of care are often expressed to me in versions of Christian idioms. I have never heard a child or an adult refer to spiritual support as emanating from spirit elders. While, as in the case of Priscilla, children may have intense relationships with their dreams of lost and deeply grieved carers, they do not appear to understand these relationships as intervening in their lives in the way that they frequently tell me that Jesus does. This of course marks a major change from the spiritual cosmologies represented in older ethnographies, where spirit elders are understood to be intensely involved in everyday life. Bourdillon described an intense relationship with spirit elders thus:

> sometime after death the deceased is settled back at home in the community and from this time on is regarded as a friendly spirit guardian to the family that survives him. The presence of these spirit guardians and their power over the lives of their descendants are so real to the traditional Shona that in many respects they remain part of the community, spirit elders whose influence remains very much alive. (Ibid.: 227)

This sense of powerful, intensely present spirit elders has not been substantiated in my fieldwork conversations with children or the adults who care for them. The waning of both the belief in, and the power of, spirit elders has been one of the topics of conversation I have had with *n'angas* who operate in Mutare. Two of these healers told me, in lament, that the power of the elders was waning. 'There has been so much suffering, so many bad things done. The spirit world is full of confusion and anger. The spirits no longer wish to care for us. The blood of the dead has angered them greatly.' As we shall see in a later chapter, this view of a serious rupture between the worlds of the living and the dead has major implications for traditional healing practices, and the ways in which people (especially children) might access them. It is not a surprising view in times of horror and extreme privation.

Care, food and eating

Care, family and kin are intimately intertwined. This is nowhere more obvious than in relation to the daily practices of care: eating, washing, cooking and the like. In the household in which Mai Takura and her sons live, finding adequate food is a daily battle. In the four years that I have known them, they have rarely had more than one week of food in storage. Most of the time they eke out small amounts over longer periods. A common meal in their home consists of *sadza* (the staple maize meal porridge), served with small amounts of relish, which is generally made from tomatoes and cabbage, rape or beans. Beans, in fact, are a luxury. Meat is unheard of. (Mai Takura, of course, remembers the relative wealth of her home when her husband was still alive and earning well, 'Then we had meat most days', she recalled.) Generally the family eat a meal of this sort once a day, mostly in the early evenings, when the children are back from school and the women back from whatever itinerant work they have been able to pursue: selling vegetables, cutting grass for the municipality, selling home-made buns. The vegetables for the evening meal are usually bought on the way home, from the money made that day. The family eat sequentially according to domestic hierarchy: Mai Takura's brother eats first, followed by the boys and then by the two adult women (who often go with less than a full share). Before school the children eat cold porridge, reserved from the night before. The adults often go without. In the summer months there may be fruit. When there has been some small financial windfall, there may be bread. Perhaps even tea with sugar.

When the family is most hard up, the women go to neighbours and ask to 'borrow' (the phrase most commonly used is *chikwereti*, on credit, meaning that it will be repaid when the donors themselves are in need and when the family have a surplus) a cup of maize meal or of beans. There are established networks of homes where one may go to seek short-term help. They are not necessarily wealthier homes. There is an understanding that hard times can be shared and that acute shortage can be ameliorated for everyone's benefit (when I have nothing, you may have a little to spare, and the tables may be turned in a few days or a week). Mai Takura and her sister-in-law go through a specific network of potential donors: the network includes the sister-in-law's brother who lives nearby, a woman who is a close friend of Mai Takura's from the market, and a few people whom she has met in the clinic or at church. The women do not ask randomly. If the members of the usual lending and receiving network have nothing, then the family goes without that day. What little there may be is usually reserved for the children, although I have often seen the adults go through the motions of pretending to eat, or saying that they have no appetite, or claiming to have eaten elsewhere during the day (even when I know this not to have been the case). If there are unexpected visitors, the visitors will be served food first. The households I have been in are extraordinary in their hospitality, given how little they have. I learnt this late, and incon-venienced families often by the poor timing of a visit. Eventually I learnt to visit at times well away from regular mealtimes, and brought food as gifts. Food cannot be refused without offence being given, although small amounts can be taken as a token (and a 'rich' visitor like me can, with acceptance, claim to have eaten enough elsewhere during the day).

I have elaborated here on practices around food in the home of Mai Takura, as the patterns are represented in other households. There are, however, variations. We have seen for example a glimpse of a meal in Priscilla's aunt's home (the incident where she was served less than the other children). I do not know how frequent an occur-rence this might be, although even older ethnographies of Shona domestic life mention the withholding of food as a common form of punishment. I do not believe that, in any of the homes I know well and have visited frequently, children are often denied food. On the contrary, it has been my repeated observation that adults, particularly women, go to extraordinary lengths to give children food before they eat.

The gender of the child may also be an important factor here. Takura and his brother have a mother, and are not expected to perform household tasks (such as cooking) that are usually associated with women's work (although they frequently do help, especially when she is ill). In the house of Isaiah's grandmother, Isaiah is also given considerable freedom from the tasks of cooking and washing. In fact his grandmother frequently complains to me that Isaiah is 'lazy' and should do more as she is getting old. But she remonstrates with him in a manner that seems to me to be half joking. At any rate, she continues to do all these things for him. She does, however, often go and stay with her widowed daughter in another part of the town, and has (in the time of my knowing her) also been to visit more distant kin in Harare. At these times, she leaves the house in the care of Isaiah, and makes it clear that she expects him to care for himself. On two of these trips to Harare, she took her daughter with her, and Isaiah was left in charge of the house and his cousins/siblings.

The labour of children

Isaiah rose to the challenge of being temporary head of the household. The cooking was done by one of his cousins/siblings, a girl of about 13. Isaiah did however ensure that there was some food in the house, and even seemed to take some pleasure in his new role. Normally, when his grandmother is away from the house, Isaiah does not like to stay there much, although he always returns to sleep. He too has a network of neighbours and friends whose houses he will visit and where he will stay until invited to eat.

In homes where the young people I know are girls or young women, they are often expected to do considerably more by way of household chores than their male counterparts. Preparing food, cooking and serving, washing dishes and pans, cleaning houses and sweeping outdoor spaces, washing clothes and caring for younger children are all tasks still considered to be appropriate for young girls. Priscilla and her female cousins are expected to do all these tasks, for themselves and for the males in the household. By contrast, boys and young men are given considerable freedom in domestic spaces, although this should not entirely conceal the fact that they too are expected to contribute to the household, even though this expected contribution is much more difficult to define. Isaiah spends large parts of the day in a nearby street market where he is well known to established stallholders and makes small amounts of money by running errands, carrying loads, and taking messages. Most of the money he makes in these ways he brings home to his grandmother, either as cash or more often in the form of groceries. He will also use the money to pay for electricity or water bills.

With these small amounts of money he tries to 'make deals'; *kukiyakiya* is the phrase he often uses for this activity.[13] It is an economic activity hard to define. It is variable. Some days it might mean lending the small amount he has to someone he knows, either for some interest or in order to participate in a larger scheme of economic activity. One day a group of boys pooled their money and bought a large container of cooking oil. The container was subsequently decanted into much smaller containers and sold at a small profit. Such activities are common among young men in urban spaces where opportunities for formal employment are scarce. To be successful the young men need to be very alert to local conditions and to have a high degree

---

[13] 'Kukiyakiya' is a common word in Zimbabwe, and could be said to refer to any activity that might or does generate income, whether in kind or cash. It reminds me of the phrase 'maak 'n plan' (from the Afrikaans: to make a plan) which I have often heard from white Zimbabweans. Again, see Jones (2010) for a much fuller account of what he has termed 'the kukiyakiya economy' in contemporary Zimbabwe.

of entrepreneurial flair. The dealing in cooking oil was the result of an awareness that, in a particular week, there was both a shortage of small containers of cooking oil and a number of potential customers looking for it.

In these matters though, Isaiah, like many of the other HIV-positive boys I know, relies heavily on the kindness of his friends. He does not seem to have the same business talent in local markets as do many of his peers. This is partly because he has a severe hearing deficit (common in HIV-positive children as a result of repeated, untreated ear infections primarily as a consequence of poor or non-existent healthcare or because there is no money to take the children to the clinic, or to buy medication). However, if he does not have the quickness of wit and sharp attention to detail that his (more able-bodied) friends do, he clearly has a gift for making and keeping friendships. It is these that sustain him, both emotionally and in terms of access to economic activity. Isaiah has learnt, though, not to speak too much about these activities, perhaps especially to people like me who offer other forms of economic potential. It took me some years to learn the arts of the marketplace from him; and, even then, he only showed me them when he was sure they would not diminish other ties between us, both economic and 'kin-like'.

Begging is another form of economic activity that I have seen boys engage in (but never girls). The plaintive beggar's call of '*batsirai*' (give me help!) is a very common sound in Zimbabwean urban spaces. Isaiah, and other boys I know, will sometimes beg (especially when circumstances are very bad or if they feel there is a reason why people may be more than usually generous, for example near Christmas or other major holidays). There is an element of the performative here. Isaiah wears his most threadbare clothes and his large, old-fashioned hearing aid (which otherwise he disdains). He has preferred places in which to beg. One is near a large bus terminus and another near a busy exit from the market. Friday evenings are often good times, especially towards the end of the month when some people have been paid. For a short while, drinking places favoured by flush diamond dealers were also popular sites for begging, offering the possibility of sudden generosity; perennially popular sites include churches on Sundays and mosques on Fridays. There is an invisible map of potential sites for begging known to these, and many other boys. Begging may also be a variable activity. Sometimes the boys will simply beg, by which I mean, choose a spot and call out or solicit for help, but more frequently it may mean washing or guarding cars, running errands and other activities associated with street children in Zimbabwean urban spaces.[14] Here the distinctions between begging and informal street work are blurred. I have, from a distance, observed Isaiah ask for money from a shopper and then, when turned down, offer to watch the car or carry goods. The money earned in these ways is small, ranging from a few cents to a few dollars.

These forms of economic activity are not available to girls because they would be seen, I think, as sex workers. Girls I know will often help their mothers, for example, if they are working in vegetable markets or selling small household items from home. (There was a thriving 'tuckshop' business in the high-density areas prior to the destruction of 'informal vending' by Operation Murambatsvina,[15] and these were generally very small retail outlets where one could buy small quantities of cheap household goods). Otherwise girls are more useful to their families if they stay home and do domestic work, before or after (or indeed, instead of) attending school. Simply moving around urban spaces can be hazardous for girls who are often propositioned, even aggressively sexually harassed, by young men, if they are unaccompanied.[16]

[14] In relation to 'street children' in Harare, see Bourdillon (1991, 1994), and (by contrast) specifically related to girls, Rurevo and Bourdillon (2003).
[15] Again, see footnote 12, p. 29, in relation to Operation Murambatsvina.
[16] Again, see Musoni 2010 though for an account of solidarity between informal vendors of both genders during Operation Murambatsvina.

Children as an investment

These then are some of the many ways in which poor, HIV-positive children can and do contribute to household economies. Of course, recurrent illness is a major obstacle here. Economic activities and useful alliances are much harder to maintain when there are periods when you are confined to your home by chest infections, diarrhoea, fever and other common illnesses. Frequent clinic appointments also disrupt these delicate balances. When I first began working in Mutare all the families I know well insisted on their children attending school, and absence from school was severely frowned upon by adults in the family. People were quite prepared to forgo the benefits that might accrue in the short term from a child's labour, when weighing it against the longer-term benefits of an educated child with a good chance of paid employment.

The collapse of the public school system in the recent past (and despite its partial resuscitation) has, I think, begun to change this perspective. Many adults still struggle quite heroically to find education for their children but are increasingly aware that managing to enrol your child in a school does not guarantee that there will be teachers to teach, as well as books and desks and chairs. There has been a boom (as I mentioned in the previous chapter) in private colleges who do have teachers and some resources, but these are considerably more expensive and generally either charge by the hour or by the subject per term. In either case the costs are prohibitive for most of the families we are considering here. Given the upheavals in education in the recent past, and its gradual deterioration prior to that, there is now a generation of children who have a very poor education, for the first time in Zimbabwe's post-colonial history.

When talking to adults in families about the decisions they have collectively made in relation to the care of HIV-positive children. I have frequently heard the phrase that the care of children is an 'investment', and that one must make it wisely. It is especially in relation to the active participation of paternal families that I have heard this. It implies a temporality of waiting. One man whom I know well told me that 'children are expensive and they take a lot from the family. It is wise to wait and see if they are going to survive before putting a lot of resources into them'. This seemed somewhat heartless to me at the time. However, if I reflect on the intensity of the daily struggle to survive, engaged in by adults and children alike, it becomes more understandable. Small children are often already settled and cared for within their mother's families. Paternal families may be too economically diminished and depleted in sheer numbers to take on additional children.

Under these circumstances, a temporality of waiting emerges. For girls there will come a time, if they live, to reconnect with paternal families if they are to marry. For boys, there will come a time that is similar but that might also be inflected with economic matters, of inheritance (in its widest sense) and perhaps even of future support. The price of the waiting is the sundering of daily connectedness, emotional support and simple affectionate acquaintance. The children have an ordeal of illness and survival to endure before families can reconfigure themselves to face an uncertain aftermath.

Care and kinship for HIV-positive children: a summary

Within Zimbabwe, in the popular media and in ordinary conversation, there is much talk of the 'breakdown' of the family. This is a series of discourses of some provenance and with some empirical basis. The physical and sexual abuse of women and children is now more widely reported than ever before, and the statistics are alarming.[17] Divorce, the dispossession of widows and various forms of familial cruelty are all staples of tabloid reporting. Popular discourse

---

[17] See, for example, www.unicef.org/Zimbabwe.

on these matters, however, also ranges over familiar territories of transnational conservatism: women abandoning their traditional roles in the domestic sphere, children becoming ungovernable, and men being immoral.[18] Morality, indeed, is the chief theme here.

One of my informants and colleagues, a pastor of great dedication, told me the following when I asked him what he thought the most urgent needs of HIV-positive children were:

> A child who is orphaned will always ask the question, why? They will be angry with their parents. They may know that their parents were immoral and thus passed a disease to them that they did not do anything to deserve. They will always wonder whether they were loved. They need to know that they were loved otherwise they will always ask, 'where is my daddy?', 'where is my mother?' Only God can answer these questions for them.

From a man who was only too well aware of the intense struggle that many children face simply in order to keep living, I found this an extraordinary answer. It is a matter of some surprise to me that even those who are well informed can privilege the moral over the simple necessities. Furthermore, in my close relationships with children over some years, I have never had a conversation in which children express anger or bitterness towards their parents who handed down the infection to them. Something else echoes in his answer, though, and that is the utter absence of crucial kin, and the longing and loss that might overtake us in trying to live on after and through such absences. Children's attachment to life struggles under conditions of great adversity against a constant ambivalence, which I have understood as a very understandable willingness to give up in the face of insurmountable odds and in the presence of the peaceful dead and a loving God. The daily recommitment to the struggle for life

---

[18] The breakdown of traditional supportive familial values has also been affected by political violence. See, for example, Jocelyn Alexander and Kudukwashe Chitofiri, 'The Consequences of Violent Politics in Norton, Zimbabwe.' *The Round Table*, Vol. 99, No. 411, 1-14 December, 2010.

is reanimated in the relationships that constitute immediate family, the desire to care and be cared for, that are constantly forged in the image of ideals about how kinship should look. In this, nostalgia and idealization are as formative as the 'traditions' handed down in language and practice. Contemporary kinship practice in Mutare, therefore, is not best understood as a static model but as a constant tension between ideals and realities in caring and being cared for. Such tensions have been noted elsewhere. For example, one of the most extraordinary accounts of kinship from an anthropologist in late 20th century kinship studies comes, I would argue, from Margaret Trawick (1990), in *Notes on Love in a Tamil Family*. Her comments are salient here:

> The main point I will try to make [in this chapter], then, is that the continuation of a particular institution [such as cross cousin marriage] may be posited, not upon its fulfillment of some function or set of functions, but upon the fact that it creates longings that can *never* be fulfilled. It is possible to see kinship not as a static form upheld by regnant or shared principles, but as a web maintained by unrelieved tensions, an architecture of conflicting desires, its symmetry a symmetry of imbalance, its cyclicity that of a hunter following his own tracks. (Trawick 1990: 152. Emphasis in the original)

4

Visible secrets
Illnesses, exposure and disclosure

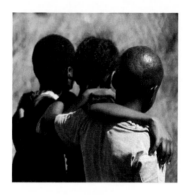

Introduction

Through a variety of landscapes, those of Mutare and its hills as
sites of sorrow and suffering, and those of familial intimacy and care
layered with grief over time, we come to a consideration of the children's experiences of illness, of the plague that is HIV. Before all
else, to a degree that frequently shocked me, HIV infection is lived
as an intense secret,[1] often even within domestic spaces where its
existence is known to all. As we shall see, the infection is everywhere
inscribed and the secret is everywhere observed. This is the case,
almost without exception, with all the children that I have come to
know, and it is a fact requiring some substantial explanation in a
country and a population where as many as 14% of the population
(and very possibly considerably more) are likely to be HIV-positive.

---

[1] It would seem indisputable that HIV is closely associated with secrecy as
a consequence of persistent and severe social stigma. See Jonny Steinberg's
(2008) richly detailed account of HIV in the Eastern Cape. For an account from
Burkina Faso, see Fabienne Hejoaka (2009). For accounts from Brazil, see João
Biehl (2005 and 2007).

'Secret' might seem the wrong word here. However ardently one may wish to conceal HIV infection, its accompanying illnesses are all too often starkly visible. Indeed many illnesses in friends, family and colleagues are quickly attributed to HIV (almost as quickly as to 'bad luck' or, worse, witchcraft). If there is a widespread wish for secrecy, it is not often effective. And yet, in the sense in which secrecy entails silence, it is precisely what appears to be at stake. The silence that surrounds HIV and its illnesses is all but absolute. One of the most poignant moments in my fieldwork was being, one early winter evening, in the home of a child as the hour approached for her to take her evening dose of antiretrovirals. Her maternal aunt, two cousins and her grandmother were all also present in their small home. The girl is not the only person in this household to be HIV-positive, or on antiretrovirals, and yet her aunt caught her eye sharply and then tapped her wrist (where her watch might have been). The girl rose and left the room, presumably to take her medicines. The rest of us continued our conversation with no mention of this silent exchange. Thereafter I became increasingly aware of the silent signals that constituted communication between carers and children about illnesses, drug dosage times and appointment reminders. In another home, the elderly grandmother's medications (for hypertension and infections) stay permanently on a small shelf next to the family Bible and an icon of the Sacred Heart, while her grandson's antiretrovirals stay wrapped in an old grocery bag beneath a pile of sleeping mats.

This chapter provides a close observation and description of children's experiences of their illness(es). Such experiences are, in part, constructed by the scale, history and form of the epidemic in southern Africa but are also inflected with the hardships consequent on Zimbabwe's failing health system and widespread poverty. Here I describe the local Mutare clinic and its patients, while also trying to be alert to older ideas about healing and illness. In this regard it is instructive that, in writing, I find it difficult to separate out matters of illness from matters of faith.[2]

Scales of illness

The delineation of the scale of HIV-related illness in Zimbabwe, as with the rest of the region, is no simple matter. Rates of infection and mortality appear to fluctuate widely between different places and regions, and over different temporalities. As the historian John Iliffe[3] has said of the epidemic in southern Africa:

> The countries of southern Africa, although infected with HIV slightly later than those further north, nevertheless overtook eastern Africa's levels of prevalence during the mid 1990s *and then experienced the world's most terrible epidemic*. By 2004 the region had 2 per cent of the world's population and nearly 30 per cent of its HIV cases, with no evidence of overall decline in any national prevalence, which in several countries exceeded 30 per cent of the sexually active population. (Iliffe, 2006: 33. My emphasis)

Firstly let us examine these statistics. In 1989 the estimates were that approximately 24% of the populations of Zimbabwe were HIV-positive and, most recently, have declined to around 14%. It is difficult to know what sense to make of these figures. In a previous chapter I have noted the extreme difficulties researchers now face in interpreting (and relying on) official Zimbabwean government statistics, or indeed of statistics produced independent of official channels within the contemporary Zimbabwean chaos. These have been too often used for narrow, parochial political interests to be considered

---

[2] It is, of course, a western cultural and intellectual distinction, dating at least to the Cartesian dichotomy of the 17th century, which attempts to hold separate the body and the mind/soul, and is deeply embedded in academic disciplines. See Marshall Sahlins (1996) for one very beautiful example of the anthropological critique of the globalizing force of the distinction.

[3] John Iliffe's (2006) history of HIV in sub-Saharan Africa is a masterly synthesis of a vast medical and public health literature.

particularly trustworthy. Furthermore the social and political climate in which data is collected must hold a direct relationship with the trustworthiness of the data then produced. As we have seen, the last decade of political crisis in Zimbabwe has seen political violence and forced displacement on an extensive scale. It has also seen the flight of a large proportion of the population into the diaspora in South Africa and elsewhere. It is entirely unclear what effects these major social disruptions have had on populations and the various projects of monitoring and measuring them. Hence figures relating to the current incidence of HIV in the Zimbabwean population must be treated with a good deal of skepticism.[4]

Again, John Iliffe is instructive on Zimbabwe's particular experience of HIV, as read through the annals of public health:

> Zimbabwe's prevalence figures are especially difficult to interpret, with wide variations between those quoted by national and international authorities, and even wider fluctuations at individual sentinel sites. The most reliable data are probably for antenatal clinic attenders in Harare. Prevalence among them was 10 per cent in 1989 and 18 per cent in 1991, both figures substantially less than in the main cities of Malawi and Zambia, but it grew further to a peak of 32 per cent in 1995 and then fluctuated around that level. Yet only 28 per cent of Zimbabwe's people were urban. The distinctive feature of its experience during the 1990s was the high level of prevalence outside the main cities, *often so high that the statistics must be treated with caution.* [Three kinds of areas were worst affected.] One contained towns on main roads close to borders, where truck drivers might socialize for several days while negotiating their way across the frontier. Beitbridge, on the South African border, recorded 59 per cent HIV prevalence in 1996, while *the figure at Mutare, near the frontier with Mozambique, reached 37 per cent in 1997.* (Iliffe, 2006: 39. My emphasis)

Figures collected in Zimbabwe in the 1990s, of course, were ob-

---

[4]   Again, see the references in footnote 12, p. 29, to the large-scale displacements within and moving out of Zimbabwe in the past decade.

tained prior to the current state of crisis but already indicated extraordinarily high levels of infection. Prior to the gradual rollout of antiretroviral treatment, beginning in the first years of the new millennium, a decline into chronic illness and eventual death was what awaited the people behind these statistics. The subsequent decade of political and economic crisis, accompanied by a collapsing healthcare delivery system and forced migration, would exacerbate the tragedy to almost unimaginable levels. My purpose in this chapter is to attend to lived experiences of children infected by HIV as a sharp humanization of the depersonalized (although already horrifying) account offered in these widely known, public health contours of the disease.

Precise figures on the scales of illness amongst children in Zimbabwe are considerably more difficult to find. However, in November 2009, the Ministry of Health and Child Welfare, in association with UNICEF (the United Nations Children's Emergency Fund) published a preliminary report from their Multiple Indicator Monitoring Survey (MIMS). The results are shocking. Under-five infant mortality was shown to have increased by 20%. The main direct causes of death were acute respiratory infections, diarrhoea, malnutrition, HIV, malaria and skin diseases.

The study also revealed that at least 79% of the orphans in the country had limited external support while the nutritional status of children had been worsened by the high poverty levels. At least 35% of the children aged under five years are stunted, 2% were wasted and 12% were underweight. Rural areas had higher levels of malnutrition than urban areas. The stunting levels in rural areas were 37% compared to 30% in urban areas. Underweight was 13% compared to 9% in urban areas (Ministry of Health and Child Welfare/UNICEF, Preliminary MIMS Report, 28 January 2009).

Here we should be acutely conscious of difficulties in understanding some of the words used above; 'orphans' being one of the more obvious.[5] The Shona languages do not have a word that might be directly translated as 'orphan'. As noted in the previous chapter, direct biological parenthood has never been equated with sole responsibility for the care and upbringing of children in regional cultures, including Shona peoples.[6] Furthermore, the report above does not relate to previous studies (that is, to data collected prior to the current crisis) so that we do not have a reliable or stable baseline with which to compare the figures.

The clinic in Mutare

Much of my personal knowledge of the effects of HIV on children in Mutare was facilitated through my close working relationship with the Paediatric Department at Mutare Provincial Hospital (as noted in my earlier discussion on methodologies). Therefore, before beginning a discussion of the experiences of HIV-related illness(es) and the ways in which these are mediated in everyday life, I want to consider the clinics at the hospital and to offer the reader a detailed description of these. My knowledge of the clinics is provided through a relatively close relationship with healthcare providers (built up over a number of years) as well as periods of close observation of the clinics, their workings and the range of patients (and illnesses) they attend to.

The children's health services, centering on the pediatric outpatient clinics, are located in the out-patient wing of the provincial hospital, located just outside of the central business district, off the main road leading to Christmas Pass and the route to Harare, and underneath a small granite kopje known as Hospital Hill. The hospital buildings, too, bear the inscriptions of history. The main in-

---

[5] See Meintjies (2005) for a parallel from South Africa.
[6] See my earlier work on children and kinship where I have also argued that parenthood in Shona cultures is not restricted to biological parents, and has never been so. Parsons (2010).

patient wing dates from the 1930s and is an elegant structure in the style usually referred to as Anglo-Indian, with arched colonnades shading deep verandahs and a red corrugated iron roof. The large out-patient wing is a modern structure, dating from the mid-1980s, and built at the height of the post-colonial government's commitment to improving healthcare delivery. The children's clinic takes place twice a week in a lower level of this wing. Probably originally a functional, clean and well-maintained building, the out-patient wing shows all the signs of the decay of public institutions suffered over the past decade and a half. Over the past four years of this study I have noticed the building gradually move from a clean and very well used space to a dirty, decaying structure with progressively fewer patients as a direct indicator of the drastically fewer services the institution is able to offer.

When I first visited the clinics in 2006, the building they were housed in greeted the new visitor with the modern hospital's sensory array of smells (disinfectant, surgical spirits and the unfamiliar), sights (strange equipment, surgical gloves, syringes) and sounds (machines, and voices, young and old, crying and whispering). By 2008 all of the above were heavily overlaid by pools of fetid rainwater, uncleaned floors and windows and eerie silences barely punctuated by few patients and even fewer staff. By that time services were almost all suspended through combinations of qualified staff leaving to join the diaspora, remaining staff engaged in industrial action (by that point many had not been paid for months), the unavailability of medical supplies and the widespread belief that the hospital was completely closed. Indeed many hospitals elsewhere in the country were closed. In Mutare some services still operated skeletally. Charity from a variety of local churches, for example, fed the few remaining in-patients.[7]

---

[7] This represents an accurate description of the situation prior to the GPA in late 2008. The GNU has managed to partially resuscitate the hospitals and clinics but not yet to standards achieved prior to 2000 and the current 'crisis'.

At the height of the recent cholera outbreak (which took place during the rainy season of 2008/2009, infecting nearly 90,000 people and killing nearly 4,000, nationally) the busiest part of the hospital, to a visitor, was the newly established International Red Cross base from which supplies for more distant rural clinics were distributed. By that stage hospital staff were surreptitiously 'borrowing' basic disinfectant from foreign Red Cross workers. The reality of state failure and indifference was unmissable.

If hygiene, drugs and staff were all in short supply (or simply absent), bureaucracy was alive and well. In this sense the presence of the state survived, perhaps even thrived. Access to the minimal services still offered required the negotiation of elaborate, layered forms of bureaucracy whose primary function appeared to be managing an intricate and burdensome system of payment. A visit to the hospital required a 'registration fee' ($4 in late 2008, $6 in early 2009). The fee was not related to services provided or received, but to single visits to the hospital. Thus, for example, an HIV-positive child might require visits within a two-week period for a range of services including a CD4 count (done through a blood test), a consultation with a healthcare provider and a trip to the pharmacy in order to obtain a new or renewed prescription for a variety of medicines. Each visit required payment of the 'registration fee'. Since some services (drugs not considered life-saving, or x-rays, for example) were no longer available in the public health system, children and their families would thereafter be referred to private health services, which were considerably more expensive. These costs cannot be underestimated in a country where over 90% of Zimbabweans are now thought to survive on less than $1 per day. Furthermore, given that many families have more than one member who is HIV-positive and in need of medical care, and in the absence of any coordination between child and adult services within the hospital, these costs can be multiplied many times over.

One of my informants, a local pharmacist working from his own pharmacy, told me that:

> Patients come to us every day with prescriptions for a range of medicines. Many will have got their antiretrovirals from the government pharmacy at the hospital, but then the doctors will have told them to take some other drugs as well. Perhaps an antibiotic for an infection, an ointment for a skin rash, a painkiller? Often all of these. The patient will quickly find out from the government pharmacy that these things are not available. The doctors are too busy to check whether the drugs they prescribe are available at an affordable price. So the patients end up in our shops. It takes a long time to help them. First they need quotes for how much the whole prescription will cost. When they find out that this is unaffordable for them, they will want to know how much each drug will cost and which would be the most important one to take. How do I advise someone? They need it all. But I have to advise and then they have to choose. They choose the painkillers. So would I. But the relief is short.

I think that it should be made clear that local staff are not primarily responsible for this dire state of affairs. Throughout 2008 the paediatric clinics operated through the quite heroic willingness of two doctors and a handful of nurses to keep working without any salaries. Furthermore, until early 2009, it was possible for patients to obtain relief from hospital registration fees although this required navigating another, quite separate government department (the Department of Social Welfare) and the process could itself be unpredictable and elaborate too. Even this potential source of relief fell away in early 2009, it is not clear why, and we have still to see what effect that will have on attendance and adherence rates.

The documentation of health care requires some description and explanation.[8] Zimbabwean children generally have two forms of health documentation: a set of hospital notes which are kept by the

---

[8] The system of documentation described here is that of government health services throughout the country.

healthcare facility (and which, in the case of HIV infection, includes an additional chart with details specific to the HIV history of the patient: when diagnosed, CD4 counts, when commenced on antiretroviral therapy (ART), for example), and an additional notebook, kept by the patient or their family, which also carries the healthcare providers' running notes on the patient's condition and the treatment(s) provided. For under-fives there is an additional chart, once again kept by families, known as a Road to Health card, which charts height and weight gain, and other early developmental milestones.

In the case of the notebook two things are striking. Firstly, they are often carefully preserved, their covers wrapped in plastic and highly decorated. Secondly, they are written obliquely since providers can never be sure who might look at them and therefore there are difficult issues of confidentiality. Thus, for example, HIV is never mentioned directly. In my experience of looking at such books HIV infection is generally recorded as 'retroviral illness' (or simply RI), or opportunistic infections (OI). Quite often there is no mention of a diagnosis at all and the reader must be able to extrapolate from the illnesses suffered or the drugs the patient is on as to what the underlying diagnosis is. Nonetheless many children I know are extremely anxious about these notebooks and their safety, although they themselves cannot understand the notes.

For example, about a year ago, Priscilla was at home when one of her cousins (mother's sister's daughter) and her school friends noticed Priscilla's clinic notebook on a table in their shared bedroom. They asked to see it. Priscilla panicked, grabbed the book and ran outside where she burnt it, seized with a fear that others might see it and 'come to know [the] secret'.[9] In this sense the notebook carries the means of being exposed, in a metaphorical although highly emotionally charged sense. It is unlikely that anyone other than a

---

[9] In this case, Priscilla (being very well known at the hospital), told staff that she had lost the book, and a new one was given to her. Of course, much detail was also lost in the change from the old notebook to the new.

professional could understand its elliptical codes, but nonetheless it remains a great source of fear and anxiety.

Observing the clinical

What constitutes the general activity of paediatric clinics such as these? I have observed their activity in detail at two separate periods. Here I summarize observations from the second of these, undertaken during the summer rainy season of 2008/2009. As noted, this was a period in which the hospital was almost entirely closed, and widely (and rightly) believed by many to have ceased functioning. In fact, in children's services, both in-patient and out-patient services were functioning. The out-patient clinic was operating two mornings a week and it was still possible for the most seriously ill to be admitted (largely through the charity of local churches who fed in-patients).[10]

During this time I attended the Wednesday morning clinic weekly for nine weeks. In this period, 250 patients were seen in this clinic, 215 of whom were HIV-positive. The great majority of the patients were returning for review, follow-up and monitoring (the paediatric services in Mutare have approximately 2,000 children registered as HIV-positive). I was told by the staff that the numbers were probably at least 15% lower than usual as a result of the crisis in the health-care delivery system, and the widely held view that the hospital was no longer operational. The numbers may indeed be significantly lower: in-patient admissions, for example, decreased more than 75% in the same period.

The following account of medical practice is specific to my observation of the Mutare hospital. Most of the HIV-positive children have been known to the clinic since birth, and have been monitored

---

[10] Again, the reader should remember that the situation has improved since the GNU although such improvements (at least in Mutare) have been slow. Most seriously the costs of using state health services remain beyond the reach of most.

since testing positive (a test that could not be deemed conclusive until the child has reached at least 18 months[11]). Prophylaxis, in the form of the antibiotic cotrimoxazole, is provided to all HIV-positive children from the time of testing positive. Antiretroviral therapy is commenced when the child's CD4 cell count has fallen below 200 (as opposed to 250-300 in much of the West, and in WHO guidelines), and the child is registered in a clinic or has some other clinical condition considered to be highly indicative of severe HIV-related illness. ART requires adherence to a strict timetable of dosages and administration. Patients' ability to comply with these standards of adherence is inculcated through a period of counselling (provided in the clinic by a nurse counsellor) and assessed, by proxy, through their adherence to cotrimoxazole. A 'failure' of adherence is a serious event that may necessitate the patient's removal from ART given that bodies can build rapid resistance to the drug under circumstances of poor or erratic adherence. The availability of antiretroviral medicines has been generally good in Mutare throughout the lifetime of my project. The medicines are made available through the government using funding from the Clinton Foundation in the USA. The drugs are generics made in India. They are manufactured in infant and 'junior' formulations and quantities although these specific preparations have not always been available and, as a result, patients and their families have had to manage complex changes in dosage depending on the availability of specific paediatric preparations.

Thus the bulk of the paediatric clinics in Mutare focus on HIV (and this is probably true nationally). There are other very common conditions, however, that both intersect with and stand apart from HIV, namely tuberculosis, malnutrition and skin infections. Tuberculosis is endemic in southern Africa and has been shown to closely shadow HIV incidence. As a category, however, it requires an x-ray for a definitive diagnosis and they were not available in the hos-

---

[11] There have been advances in early paediatric testing and a definite diagnosis can now be obtained much earlier.

pital at the time of my observations. Standard drug therapies for TB are known to interfere with antiretroviral medications. Doctors in Mutare prefer to treat TB prior to starting ART. Malnutrition (including forms of chronic under-nutrition) is widespread in Zimbabwe. One of my informants, a paediatrician, tells me that as many as a third of Zimbabwean children show signs of poor nutrition. The signs are very clear in the clinic: stunting, thinness, apathy and weakness are all distressingly common. Clinical syndromes of various forms of malnutrition (kwashiorkor, marasmus and pellagra, for example) are relatively common and distressing for both patients and professionals. The following is taken from my field notes after one clinic:

> The horror came at the end in the form of Abigail, a 12-year-old girl who looked to have been lifted directly out of an Oxfam horror video from Ethiopian famine. Utterly skeletal, huge eyes, looking as though a single breath of wind might finish her off. She was with her grandmother from Manica Bridge: a big, stout woman who answered all questions briskly and comprehensively. It was hard to see whether there was much affection between them. Abigail herself sat slightly askew, very agitated, hands fluttering on the protruding bones at her neck, no words, no sounds, and no sustained eye contact with anyone in the room. Not crying. How I wanted her to be crying. It is the silent, terribly sick children, so seemingly indifferent to their fates that most distress me. She will be admitted. [The doctor] is not hopeful but invokes his favourite category of the Lazarus figure.[12] The grandmother seemed neither relieved nor, indeed, much interested. But then again she has five other children at home, one of whom had

---

[12] The Gospel of John: 11: 1-44 gives the Christian account of Jesus miraculously raising a man named Lazarus from the dead. By invoking the biblical story of Lazarus, the doctor suggests that miraculous healing is always possible despite his professional judgment that recovery is unlikely. This is a good example of the ways in which strong Christian beliefs imbue much of everyday life in Zimbabwe. The clinic often begins with staff prayer, as do many mundane meetings in Zimbabwe generally.

chronic TB. [About three-quarters of the HIV children have TB, or pneumonia, or severe skin rashes.] I want someone else in the room to weep with me, or be horrified. (Fieldnotes)

One of the most widespread afflictions seen in the clinic is skin rashes and subsequent secondary infections. They are especially common in HIV-positive children and are an especially visible form of vulnerability and infection. Skin disorders range from fungal infections (ringworm for example) to scabies and infected sweat glands. The severe itchiness of the infestations oftens cause raw patches which then become infected with secondary staphylococci, leading to weeping sores and ever widening and deepening cycles of infection and re-infection. Rashes are often to be found on heads and behind major joints, leading to poor flexibility and mobility. Weeping wounds attract flies, and attention. Medications are not available for these conditions (they are not life-threatening)[13] and frequently children must endure long periods of suffering and significant scarring and disfigurement.

From my knowledge of the health services available to children in Mutare I would say that sustained treatment, albeit in very limited forms, is available to those who have some resources, not the least of which is the ability to interact effectively with complex bureaucratic systems and access to (or money for) transport to and from hospital, and for registration fees. HIV-positive children might receive continuous, professional care within certain limits. The limits include acceptance of the limits of care. Access to medications is dependent on the generosity of donors and premised on the category 'life saving', which might be highly problematic (for example, children with severe skin infections cannot access appropriate and effective

---

[13] By which I mean, such medications are not available in the hospital pharmacy where medications are free. Such medications are available in private pharmacies but at costs that would be prohibitive for most Zimbabweans (a standard anti-fungal cream in a private pharmacy in Zimbabwe would probably cost around $6).

medications even though the infections and their consequent disfigurement may well be a major factor working against sustained adherence to antiretroviral drugs, and the secondary infections may become life-threatening.) Generally, attention to children's most urgent and pressing medical needs is all that can be managed by very hardworking and under-resourced staff. One consequence is that psychological issues receive little or no attention. I have never heard a conversation in the clinics about a child that relates to grief, depression or trauma. This is remarkable given the high utility and widespread valence of such ideas in many similar clinics elsewhere in the world (but, perhaps, particularly in the West).

The marks of torment and illness

The difficulty with a phrase like 'chronic illness' (a common contemporary moniker of 'living with HIV') is that it fails to capture, or communicate, the random and unpredictable nature of HIV-related illness(es). As we shall see, it may also be inaccurate. It has long been a truism of HIV literature that people do not die of HIV infection, but rather that a severely weakened immune system renders them vulnerable to a multiplicity of illnesses. It is worth reflecting on what these might entail. The children I know have suffered from forms of diarrhoea, chest infections, ear infections, eye infections, multiple different forms of skins infections (manifesting on different parts of the body), tuberculosis, pneumonia, and malaria. Some of these ailments (such as diarrhoea, stomach pain and nausea) are often associated by the children with the drugs they take, and others (like malaria and tuberculosis) are endemic in the community and are not experienced as being particularly related to being HIV-positive.

Tinashe was a 13-year-old boy when I met him in 2005. He lives with his mother and younger brother. All are HIV-positive. His father died six years before we met. Tinashe has fairly close relationships with his father's family who live some 20kms outside of Mutare in an area known as Zimunya (but his mother does not). He had just started taking antiretrovirals although his mother has been taking them for some two years. Tinashe was very small for his age, and looked about eight years old when I met him. The family are very poor. They live in the high-density area of Dangamvura where his mother struggles to make ends meet by brewing and selling beer from the one room she rents in a house. Tinashe and his mother have a very difficult relationship. His mother tells me that he steals from her and often runs away (going to stay at his father's mother's house in Zimunya).

Tinashe is never easy to talk to. Besides being small, he is a very quiet and elusive boy. Throughout 2005 and 2006 he suffered from a severe skin rash that probably started as a case of ringworm on his scalp, arms and legs. No medication and much scratching caused raw, weeping skin that was soon plagued by a secondary infection. For long periods of time Tinashe was very distressed by it. He wore oversized clothing to hide his limbs, and a large hat pulled well down to hide his head, that failed to hide the problem and, instead attracted attention to him – clouds of flies were attracted to his head, with or without a hat – and the abrasion of cloth against raw skin was itself very uncomfortable. He went weeks unable or unwilling to attend school. The infection took months to abate. It was clear that Tinashe and his mother lived with a considerable degree of tension and discomfort in their relationship, exacerbated by cramped poor surroundings, constant anxiety about money and food and their respective illnesses.

In early 2008, Tinashe was again plagued by a severe skin infection, similar to the previous one and affecting the same areas. In addition he developed a severe infection in his right eye, which was swollen and mostly closed for a period of over three months. He could barely see and he found his scalp and eye intolerably painful. He began to spend increasingly long periods of time at his father's mother's house. Staying at her house meant that he could not attend clinic appointments. He seemed to be continuing with his antiret-rovirals, which he obtained from a local clinic. He told me on one occasion when we met at the group that he saw no point in going to the clinic at the hospital where he felt he received neither treat-ment for, nor understanding of, the health problems that most tor-mented him. 'They just tell me to wash my head and shave my hair and to wait,' he said, in both despair and anger; 'they have nothing to help me'. Then he criticized his mother for being too docile at the clinic and at the same time for not spending money on medications from private pharmacies (I was aware, as I think he was too, that the prices of these medications were simply beyond his mother's means). Despair demanded a bald statement, words that match harsh feel-ings. Tinashe felt that the care offered by the clinic was unrelated to his sufferings.

Enduring illness(es)

It is not always particular illnesses that mark one out socially as likely to have HIV, but the number, range and repetitiveness of illnesses, as well as other physical forms of presentation (especially thinness). When I have asked people in Mutare, as I often have, whether it was possible to tell HIV-positive people by appearance, everyone agreed that it was and I was given the following characteristics: being very thin, coughing a lot, being very pale, having red and cracked lips, having sparse hair, and being sick a lot. The children are very aware of these characteristics and will actively seek ways to avoid them. As we have seen previously, some of the children in the group match many of these descriptions, others do not.

Many children, though, however much and fervently they may wish to hide their status as infected, carry the inscriptions of ill-ness on their bodies in obvious ways. Priscilla, for example, as stated before, is very thin and very small for her age. (Now aged 19, Pris-cilla looks as if she is 14 or perhaps younger). Here we should note, however, that stunting in itself is unlikely to be entirely attributable to HIV infection.[14] Malnutrition and chronic under-nutrition are common in Zimbabwean children under the age of 12. A paediatrician informant estimates that as many as a third of children in Zimbabwe demonstrate a significant degree of stunting as a consequence of poor nutrition. We also know, of course, that chronic poor nutrition in early childhood may lead to significant cognitive delays and difficulties that are hard to assess given the simultaneous collapse of public schooling (and of educational psychology services within the state education system).

However, to return to Priscilla, we might also note that her hair is sparse (and its scarcity makes it difficult for her to effect the most fashionable weaves that other girls her age do). Her skin is mottled and scarred as a direct consequence of frequent skin infections so that her HIV status cannot be kept hidden however fervently she might wish to conceal it. In her physical appearance she fulfills most of the prevailing stereotypes of what someone with 'AIDS' would look like.

In my time in Mutare, there have been no anti-fungal drugs available at the General Hospital. In fact, the General Hospital has been reduced to only having drugs that are considered 'life saving' (antiretrovirals, antibiotics, drugs for TB) and these drugs are made available through the generosity of large, transnational NGOs. The hospital cannot provide any other forms of medication, including painkillers (except for paracetamol). Its nutritional supplements are only available for infants.

Beside the widespread problems associated with fungal and secondary skin infections, there are other less obvious problems. One of the largest of these is the level of hearing loss associated with HIV infection as a result of repeated, untreated ear infections. It

[14] Again, see the national rates for stunting and malnutrition as discussed earlier in the chapter. Ministry of Health and Child Welfare/UNICEF, Preliminary MIMS Report, 28 January 2009.

is common for children to develop ear infections characterized by irritation, and an oozing of pus and mucus. They are not ailments likely to elicit rapid recourse to medical care by families (or to justify the costs of using healthcare). Health professionals whom I have spoken to, confronted with these forms of ear infection, simply advise carers to keep the ear dry by swabbing it frequently, although they acknowledge that there is a high level of hearing loss amongst HIV-positive children. One paediatrician estimated, in conversation with me, that up to 20% of HIV-positive children have a 'significant degree of hearing loss'.[15] We have seen the instantiations of such forms of deafness in the life of Isaiah. A further way in which hearing loss has profound effects on the lives of some children is their poor academic achievement in an already failing education system. Hearing loss, stunting and skin infections (new and old), in addition to regular bouts of acute illness, combine to make it difficult for children to take advantage of what education is available.

Unlikely survivors

Almost all of the children have been HIV-positive since birth. Many have been registered in the Mutare paediatric service since birth. Nicholas is the only one who is likely not to have been infected from birth (we shall meet him in more detail in a later chapter) but to have become infected (probably) through adolescent sexual activity. It is a remarkable fact in itself since, prior to the availability of antiretroviral treatment and of prevention of mother-to-child transmission programmes, most children born HIV-positive were expected to be dead by the age of five. How they have survived is not known. One way in which the uncertainty about likely survival has affected children, their families and healthcare providers has been through a very problematic relationship to disclosure.

[15] I am not sure what, medically speaking, constitutes 'significant' in degrees of hearing loss.

Consider the following account taken, again, from my fieldnotes:

> Today [a doctor] asked my advice about one of his patients in the children's clinic. His dilemma concerns an 18-year-old boy who the doctor has treated since infancy, and who he has known to be HIV-positive since then. Now it is time to transfer the boy to an adult clinic and at this point [the doctor] 'realizes' that he has never had an open conversation about being HIV-positive with his patient 'because I was never sure he was going to survive and after a certain point I began to assume that he must know' ... [A]fter some weeks I heard that [the doctor] had openly discussed the boy's diagnosis with him and had been shocked by [the patient's] very distressed response, 'I never knew', he had said. (Fieldnotes)

The account raises serious questions about the nature and quality of care children receive, and the absolute elision of attention to their emotional wellbeing. It is frighteningly clear that healthcare providers are struggling with disclosure to infected children. Families also struggle with when and how to tell children of their HIV status. Adults, who care for the children from our group, many of them themselves HIV-positive, tell me that their greatest concern is to avoid causing children shock or distress. 'If she knows,' said one carer of her 13-year-old charge, 'she might become disheartened and unable to go on. She will think too much.' (Here the word is *kururisa*/lit: to think too much). This is a complicated dilemma. We should remember that most of the children have been known to be HIV-positive since birth and, therefore, at that stage far too young to understand their health status. As a child grows, and outlives the immediate threat of death, carers must make decisions about when to formally 'tell' children about their status or, in my experience, more commonly, hope that knowledge will simply dawn on them in other ways. The case of the 18-year-old I have cited above would suggest that at least some young people may remain unaware for extended periods (although then I would be intrigued to know what sense they have made of an entire childhood marked by frequent trips to clinics, close medical monitoring and multiple illnesses[16]).

As I have described in Chapter 2, when I first began running the children's 'psychosocial' support group I asked all the children who came, when alone with each, what was wrong with them. Only one answered by saying she had HIV, the rest mentioned tuberculosis or pneumonia. I had been told by medical staff that each had been told of their diagnosis in the clinic. I knew they had received strong messages from members of their families never to discuss or disclose their status, and the injunctions were taken in absolute and all-encompassing ways. I have wondered whether there was a hiatus of sorts between knowing and voicing. It seems to me that the children have had very few situations in which they have been able or allowed to practice, as it were, the performances of disclosure. The group has been useful to them, very slowly, as a place in which it is possible to speak of HIV.

The fear of openly voicing HIV infection relates to associated fears of what might happen as a consequence of exposure. I use the word 'exposure' here to point to the social devastation that might ensue from the secret of my infection becoming known. Many of the children have had experiences of stigma, shame, mockery and even threatened violence. They have also heard stories from and of each other in these situations. For example, some six months ago, Priscilla was walking to the church where the group meets near the centre of Mutare. It was during the time when schools were not functioning and, perhaps as a result, many young people were bored and often to be seen on the streets. Close to the church, Priscilla passed a group

[16] See footnote 1, p. 92, for a previous discussion of the nature of the 'secrecy' that surrounds HIV in which I suggested that secrecy is primarily a response to social stigma. This incident however suggests a much more complex relationship between social and psychological forces. Doctors and nurses (and families) avoid frank discussion, *consciously or unconsciously*, and all actors share silence. It also suggests that disclosure is seen as a single event rather than an extended process, in which different levels of knowledge are given to children as they mature.

of four or five adolescent boys who began to both mock her, saying that she was thin and ugly (and therefore someone who 'obviously had AIDS'), and threaten her with rape and a beating. Priscilla was at first tart in response but rapidly became more fearful. One of the boys pulled her sweater and she ran for the shelter of the church. After the incident she was very distressed and afraid of walking alone through the town. Nor is this Priscilla's only experience of social exposure. She has endured incidents at school where she has been repeatedly taunted by older girls for having 'AIDS'.

Sociality and the clinic

It is not, I think, that the healthcare professionals in the clinic fail to see the pressing nature of children's more immediate infections but rather than they know there is little they can do to ameliorate them. It is also possible that, faced with their ineluctable uselessness, professionals tend to sound dismissive when talking to carers and patients about symptoms such as skin, ear and eye infections. I think, however, that children often interpret the stance as being indifferent to their more immediate problems, and that they therefore feel diminished and rejected. In a similar fashion it is intriguing to me to notice that a similar gulf exists when it comes to the children's experiences of the most distressing side effect of antiretrovirals, which is that they make you hungry.

We have seen in the previous chapter an incident in the life of Priscilla where, in the context of feeling herself to be a burden in the house of her mother's sister, she is acutely conscious of her increased hunger and her justified fear that, acting on this hunger by eating more, will mark her out as greedy in the domestic terrain she struggles to negotiate. The children have a very diffident relationship with this property of antiretrovirals in contexts of limited food and many mouths. An increased appetite is, of course, one of the benefits of antiretrovirals, restoring weight loss and building physical reserves against future infection. Nonetheless children living in poverty appear to experience it as a problem.

Embarrassment concerning what is felt to be an inappropriate hunger is contrasted with nausea, the common side effect of cotrimoxazole (the prophylactic antibiotic). The children I know dislike the drug intensely and have very negative associations with taking it, even though many of them took it for extended periods (as we noted earlier). It is the drug used for prophylaxis in all children known to be HIV-positive prior to their being deemed sick enough to start antiretrovirals. It would seem to me, trying to think about the drugs from the perspective of children who have taken both for long periods, that both drugs appear to be somewhat disconnected from their everyday experience. This is not to say that they are not aware, to various extents, that the drugs have saved their lives but rather that the benefits of the drugs are measured within the contingency of everyday pressures, be they pressing illness or a strained domestic atmosphere. To map the aims of the clinic onto the experiences of children, both within their own bodies and in their family worlds, produces a sense of a social field of depth in which it becomes increasingly difficult to think of adherence (or non-adherence) in simple or linear ways.

It also becomes difficult to think of the social as fully separate from the individual. To return to the problem of the extraordinary secrecy that surrounds HIV, I want to consider the clinic's own waiting room as emblematic here. I have already discussed statistics from the clinics, which demonstrate that they are busy and that a majority of their patients attend in order to receive treatment for HIV and its related disorders. Likewise, we have seen examples of the intense secrecy in which HIV is held, even within families where more than one person is infected. The busy waiting rooms of the clinics are, thus, an interesting study in both secrecy and sharing. Patients and their families are adept at reading different forms of documentation and physical ailments and symptoms. I think it is clear to most long-time users of the hospital's services what these differences point to. And, of course, over two-thirds of a waiting room on any given day will be HIV-positive. However, my observation of waiting rooms is that they are generally silent with the exception of the crying of very young children and the brisk directions of the nurses (who weigh and measure each child on arrival).

The waiting room is a long room, almost like a very broad corridor, with smaller rooms for doctors, nurses and administrators leading off it. It is dominated by rows of long wooden benches on which children and their various carers sit while waiting to see the doctor. Nurses know the children and families very well and, in my experience, have a prodigious memory for names, ages, family details, and schools attended. The queue is strictly observed by all and politeness rules. If a child or carer is called away from the queue, their neighbour will carefully hold their place, and often hold their documentation too. What it took me longer to discover, though, is that patients and carers also have prodigious memories for other patients and carers. These memories run from clinic to clinic but are also refreshed in other spaces: markets, schools, buses, and neighbourhoods. Against the extraordinary silence and stilted formality of the waiting room, some other kinds of sociality slowly emerge. As we saw in the previous chapter, Mai Takura has a tightly knit circle of relatives and friends to whom she can turn to borrow food at times of extreme shortage. One of these women is someone who Mai Takura first saw in the clinic waiting room, subsequently saw on buses to their shared neighbourhood and with whom she very slowly developed a friendship. Extraordinarily, though, Mai Takura tells me that she and her friend have never openly discussed their visits to the clinic or the illnesses of their children. Friendship and close support has grown in a context of shared secrecy and social circumspection.

Ritual and healing

Much of the material and thoughts here concern the western clinic and its treatments, and how the treatments impact on children's experiences of their own ill health. It is instructive to consider how this web of relationships and practices sits, as a template, on other ideas about illness and healers. A body of such ideas is to be found in relation to older Shona ideas about healers, patients and illnesses.

In an older Shona cosmology, illness is the principal symptom that points to a disturbance between the living and the dead.[17] The disturbance may be a sign of unease and discord between living persons and the spirits of their ancestors (*midzimu*/plural), or may indicate the work of evil as personified through the actions of witches and sorcerers (*varoyi*/plural). In either case, the illness is thought to require two responses: a divination by a *n'anga* to diagnose the nature of the rift between living and dead (and thereby to ascertain the ritual activity required to put it right) or to identify the likely witch, and a treatment (either through the herbalism of traditional medicine or the treatment of western medicine, or both) to allay the symptoms of the present illness and to cure it. Here it is important to note that ancestral spirits are those of a family (and a kinship), and the family member whose illness is the index of discord between the living and the dead may not be the individual (or group of individuals) whose actions (or inactions) have angered the spirits. A consultation with a traditional healer is not an affair for the individual. As Bourdillon notes, 'In a matter of some moment the consultation becomes a family affair usually arranged and financed by the family head. If someone in the family is seriously ill, he will not be able to travel himself to a distant diviner. So a delegation including, or at least representing, the family head is made responsible for the consultation' (1976: 152). It is my experience that children are often

---

[17] See Holleman (1952) and Bourdillon (1976).

detached from their father's families, and that this mode of consultation essentially prohibits consulting traditional healers; a fact that we shall return to shortly.

In the grammar of traditional healing, the most effective healing requires the healer to be a conduit between the living and the dead which is a state achieved through possession by the healing spirit. The possession may happen during the consultation, or may come in the form of dreams, before or after meeting the patient. The healer is believed to have access to information about the patients that do not require eliciting information from the patient and their families during the consultation. The performance of consultation thus does not allow for the direct eliciting of information. One of the measures of a good healer is that they are able to diagnose ailments through their access to the realm of the spiritual. As Bourdillon puts it, 'When he has shown his clients that he is able to discover the cause of their errand without having to be told, they can consult his oracles with confidence' (1976: 152). Here is an interesting difference with forms of western medicine where, by way of strong contrast, the healer must elicit detailed and extensive information from the patients and their families.

It might be illuminating to think back to the experience of Mai Takura that we encountered in the previous chapter. When her husband became seriously ill, his family took him to a *n'anga* in Chipinge.[18] The *n'anga* decided through divination that Takura's father was being plagued by an ancestral spirit who wished him to become a medium and a healer. Takura's father, of course, died before he could act on this information. Since his death, and his family's dispossession of his widow, Mai Takura and her sons have not been back to a *n'anga*. At times she explains this as a consequence of her deeply held Christian beliefs, at other times she explains it as one of

[18] Healers from far away are often considered less influenced by local knowledge (a good thing) and healers from remote places, such as Chipinge or Mozambique, are often considered more potent.

the negative consequences of her sundered relationship with her late husband's family. 'It is not my place to consult my husband's family's spirits,' she tells me; 'for this I would need the help of my mother-in-law or my husband's brothers.' In this way the combination of forms of patrilineal kinship and their imbrications in the grammars of traditional healing effectively exclude Mai Takura and her sons from seeking help in these domains, and the exclusion is rendered in a Christian vein as a Christian duty.

Mai Takura does have a deep knowledge of local herbal pharma-copeia, which she learnt from her mother when still a girl. One day, sitting in the courtyard of the church, I asked her whether she ever used herbs to treat either herself or her sons. She explained that she was anxious about doing so since various doctors had warned her of potentially negative interactions with other medicines. However, around the bench we sat on, she was able to point out to me many common plants with medicinal properties (to control diarrhoea, to promote digestion, to calm fever, for example). I suggested that she should feel confident about her own knowledge and skill. Since then I have noticed that her sons seem less susceptible to minor infections.[19]

In the course of the study, I have come to know a number of tra-ditional healers working in Mutare. Of the five I have come to know quite well, all but one are spirit mediums. The remaining one is pri-marily a herbalist although she does have a tutelary spirit who, in her dreams, instructs her as to the appropriate preparations that will be most beneficial to particular patients. Of the spirit mediums, three are possessed by the spirits of ancestors who were themselves heal-

---

[19] I am not suggesting here that the two are connected, and certainly not on a causal level. I am pointing out a difference in ideas and practices in the prac-tice of biomedicine in Zimbabwe (and much of the global south) and wealthier (northern/western) contexts. Many HIV-positive people in wealthier, cultur-ally various societies make very active use of both biomedicine and alternative therapies.

ers while the fourth is possessed by a *mashave* spirit (an alien spirit). All but one also claim to be Christians. A combination unthinkable, for example, in the relatively clear-cut worlds of older ethnographies, where traditional and Christian were clearly demarcated and mutually exclusive, although it seems somewhat unclear how their Christian communities would feel about these complex cross-connections, if they know about them.

All the healers, as I described in the previous chapter, speak with some anguish about unprecedented turmoil in spirit worlds as a direct consequence of the violence and suffering of the past decade of Zimbabwean crisis. They point to mass violence (the Gukurahundi massacres, the depredations of Operation Murambatsvina, the social displacements which have led to situations where 'people don't know where their ancestors' graves are') as generating serious ruptures between living and dead, and suggest that the dead have grown unwilling to help the living anymore. One of the *n'angas* told me that his clients had grown old and that people were now less inclined to consult him about their children's illnesses, although this did not seem borne out to me on the days he invited me to observe his work.

I have also come to know a 'prophet', a healer from one of the independent Zionist churches. The 'prophet' is by far the busiest of these healers and, I think, on some days as busy as the clinics.

Christian healing

There are a variety of African independent churches, dating back to the early years of the 20th century, with a great many followers. The *vapostori* (apostles), with their shaved heads, staffs and white robes are a very common Zimbabwean sight, both urban and rural. There is an extensive literature on the churches in the region (Daneel 1971, Bourdillon 1976, Comaroff and Comaroff 1991). Healing rituals among 'prophets' differ from those amongst *n'angas*, primarily in the absolute rejection of the powers of the spirits of the dead. This is not to say that such spirits are held not to exist, which they most definitely are, but that the power of the Christian Holy Spirit is held to be more powerful, and readily available to those who have received its Gifts (one of the principal of which is that of healing). Bourdillon gives the following account of Apostolic healing practices:

> Diagnosis by a prophet follows closely the patterns of diagnosis by traditional diviners, although the insight of the prophet is supposed to come from a different source than that of a traditional diviner. Both types of diviner attribute disease to conflict with spiritual powers or to conflicts within the community supported by witchcraft. But the two types differ radically in their prescriptions for a cure: whereas traditional diviners recommend appeasement of the spiritual powers, prophets base their therapy on the belief that the power of the Christian God can overcome all other power.[20] (1976: 304)

The children and adults from our group claim never to have consulted a *n'anga* with their families but all of them readily admit to receiving a wide variety of faith-healings. Such healings are not only the preserve of the African Independent churches. The newer charismatic and Pentecostal churches are extremely active sites for the practice of the laying-on of hands and the invocation of the healing powers of the Holy Spirit. Many of the forms of faith-healing are, in my observation, now shorn of all ritual trappings. Workers in the (Pentecostal) church office will pray for children and their carers, and lay on hands, with no more ado than they would approach the most mundane of tasks. In the next chapter we shall examine in detail the nature of churches and their intense relationship with

[20] 'Apart from appeasing the cause of illness, traditional healers provide medicinal treatment to remove the symptoms. Prophets generally reject all medicines and claim to rely solely on the power of the Holy Spirit for their cures. They do, however, use symbolic instruments which find parallels in the traditional treatment of disease. Thus a patient may be instructed to inhale the smoke from burning shreds of sanctified paper in order to drive out a spirit; sanctified needles may be used to remove evil blood from a patient ... and sanctified water is a general protection against evil.' (Bourdillon 1976: 304)

ideas of illness, suffering and healing. These forms of healing are radically democratized and fully accessible, with a prior or simultaneous conversion and confession of Christian faith.

Summary

The chapter proceeds from the idea that HIV infection is not always experienced as a chronic illness but rather often as unpredictable exposure to multiple, random illnesses. In the course of the argument I have examined the processes and relational dynamics at play in children's 'coming to know' of their diagnosis, and the consequences it entails, including voicing such knowledge. Many HIV-infected children in our group are brought up within family atmospheres often constituted by intense secrecy which becomes increasingly untenable in the face of multiple AIDS-related bereavements as well as the multiplying inscriptions of illnesses on their bodies (in the forms, primarily, of stunting, hearing loss and disfigurements).

While secrecy is fiercely adhered to, it is mediated in social spaces such as clinics. The clinic is itself precariously constituted and sustained in the failing health system (and indeed the failing state), and has few remaining powers. The availability of antiretrovirals and basic antibiotics, and the frail continuity of known health professionals are chief amongst these. The pharmaceuticals are experienced differently by children, and their effects measured against the more immediate demands of their social worlds. There are other forms of social support present here: in the rituals of the waiting room and the informal support systems that arise between children and their caregivers; a solidarity of 'those who know'. Such social structures bear the weight of passing on knowledge and skill (to find food, to bear with both hunger and nausea, to resist social exclusion, amongst much else) in the face of the overwhelming odds against survival that currently, persistently and perniciously, constitute much of the Zimbabwean social landscape.

5

If I had faith
Churches, spirits and healing

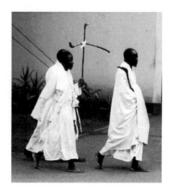

Introduction

Within the landscapes of Mutare, as one particular urban and social configuration within contemporary Zimbabwe, we have seen how the forms of the HIV epidemic, and their intersections with historical processes (perhaps most immediately the post-colonial crisis), have brought specific forms of suffering and endurance to HIV-positive children. These forms of suffering are embedded in the decimation of families, the pervasive grief that dominates domestic terrains, and the changes thereby wrought to ideas and experiences of 'ideal' kinship, and the practices of care that continue in the remnants of families. In particular, children's experiences of illness, and their vulnerability to ever more illness, is in part mediated by the local children's health services which persist in limited forms through the tenacity of a few healthcare providers.

The local clinics are able to provide forms of continuous care, constructed around ideas and practices of what constitutes the 'life-saving', although many children find their most pressing healthcare issues unattended to in this dialectic. The visible signs of their illnesses are starkly manifest despite their deep efforts to maintain absolute secrecy in the face of the potentially devastating consequences of social exposure. The promises of western medicine, undermined by a severe lack of resources and the indifference of a failing state, continue a complex relationship with older forms of healing (and attendant understandings of misfortune) that have been usually rendered as 'traditional'. At play here are a series of powerful conceptual binaries: 'traditional/modern', 'superstition/science' and 'Christian/pagan', for example. In a number of ways these binaries obscure persistent relationships of co-existence and interpenetration, as we have seen in relations between traditional healing and western medicine. Richard Werbner (a scholar who has attended to religious transformation in southern Africa over the *longue durée*) notes:

> The modernist paradigm of religious change takes a number of things for granted, all of which are questionable ... the Christian religion is assumed to be in time, revelatory of the past, prophetic for the future and devoted to the Crucified God who intervenes in history, ultimately through the mysticism of suffering. All that leaves 'traditional religion' caught in the other half of the dichotomy – the traditional is thus unchanging, static, timeless, out of time and out of history .... Against that, it is modernity alone that is inscribed with the hallmark of the highly autonomous individual; modernity alone that sows doubt; modernity alone that suffers from secularization; and it is modernity alone that bears our burden – angst and alienation. (Werbner 1997: 312)

In Werbner's account, our understanding of religious experience is hampered as much by our paradigms as by our lack of specificity. The theoretical oppositions of 'traditional' versus 'Christian' versus 'modern' are themselves obstacles to a fuller understanding of religious experiences and formations in southern Africa, and their social entailments (including their political consequences). It is clear that religious practice in the everyday combines elements of all of the above.

In this chapter I will examine in detail the nature of religious practice[1] in relation to survival in the face of dire poverty, and of illness, suffering and anticipated death. If the clinics, and less socially obvious forms of healing, mediate children's experiences of their illnesses, and their vulnerabilities, then institutional forms of religious practice (and underlying spiritual belief) can also be understood to mediate experience. In particular, Christian churches, old and new, take on these tasks but, as we shall see, yet older forms of understanding and practice persist. The relationships between 'traditional' beliefs and practices, and an intense engagement with various forms of Christianity, are not best described in the ambit of 'either/or'.

It is instructive that it is a difficult task to demarcate distinctions between healing and spirituality, and therefore to mark a break between a chapter that attends to healing and clinics and a chapter that attends to spirituality. Writing in 1976, Michael Bourdillon had this to say about Shona attitudes to illness and healing:

> On the one hand, the Shona are often terrified by serious illness; on the other hand, they often appear indifferent to the outcome of treatment [*this is a statement originally attributed by Bourdillon to Michael Gelfand's writing in 1944*] received from doctors of western medicine and to have no incentive to fight an illness. The reason behind these two attitudes lies in the belief that serious or abnormal illness, like anything out of the ordinary, is caused by spirits, perhaps angered spirits, or by witchcraft or sorcery. Until the ultimate cause of the trouble is discovered and appeased or overcome, there remains the frightening possibility of further trouble, and it is hopeless to expect complete relief from the present affliction. According to Shona belief, western medical treatment can only alleviate symptoms of abnormal illness, or at best it can cure the present illness, but it remains use-

---

[1] By stressing religious *practice* here, I am also pointing out that it is very difficult to study *belief*. What people say they believe may differ markedly from their actual practices. It is only the latter, however, that are available for observation.

less against the original cause of an illness which can always strike again. (1976: 149)

As I remarked in the previous chapter, amongst urban Shona people living in Mutare, and suffering from HIV (and its related illnesses), it seems that there is a level of indifference, apprehension and avoidance to the healing practices and rituals offered by traditional healers and spirit mediums. We have examined a number of reasons why this may be the case: for example, the absence of appropriate kin to approach *n'anga*, and uncertainties about interactions between western pharmaceuticals and *mushonga* (ritual herbal treatments). In addition, however, there are now widespread beliefs and anxieties[2] about the demonic nature of all spiritual life and practice that is not specific to (and specifically condoned by) those forms of the spiritual sanctioned by varieties of Christian churches, and their attendant theologies.

Language alerts us to a subtle but crucial difference in relation to faith and its practices in Zimbabwe. The Shona word for faith is *chitendero* (which might also be translated as 'teachings'); however, in my daily experience, it is a word little used. By contrast, people use the verb *kunamata* (to pray) frequently both in the sense of their actual religious practices as well as an indicator of the specific affiliations to which they subscribe. Thus to say *'tinamata kwaRoma'* (we pray as Roman Catholics) implies both that we consider ourselves to be Catholics as well as indicating the types of prayers and other devotional practices that may be entailed (such as the use of the rosary or of iconography). It tells us that religious belief is understood as a practice, and as a group practice, rather than as only (or even) a matter of individual conviction. Fundamentally though, for all my informants, children and adults alike, there is a sincere and intense effort to be good Christians.

---

[2] For an account of the relationship between 'new' Christianities and anxiety, see Webb Keane (2006).

Churches in Mutare

Christianity is the dominant religion of Zimbabwe, in all its many splendoured versions. In the national consultations on a new constitution in 2000 (the event that most immediately preceded the subsequent descent into violence, chaos and misgovernance that has characterized the past decade), it is a little remarked fact that a motion to declare Christianity as the 'official religion' of Zimbabwe was only very narrowly defeated. In fact it was probably only defeated because that version of a new constitution was so thoroughly defeated in a subsequent referendum primarily as a rejection of unlimited terms of office for unpopular leaders. This is remarkable given that forms of Christianity had only been widely disseminated in the country since the advent of colonialism in the late 19th century, although there had been a much earlier (and tragic) visit by Portuguese Jesuits to the court of the Mwene Mutapa.[3] (Although here it should be noted that anthropologists working elsewhere, for example, Joel Robbins, 2004, in Papua New Guinea and Webb Keane, 2007, in Sumbun, Indonesia, have documented even more rapid and absolute mass conversions to Christianity).

As recently as 1976, Bourdillon estimated that as few as 17% of Zimbabweans had an allegiance to one or other of the mainstream Christian churches, and that a further 8% had an allegiance to one or other of the African independent churches.[4] The figures may sug-

[3] For a more substantial account of the ill-fated visit (1560-61) of the Portuguese Jesuits, led by Father Silveira, to the court of the Mwene Mutapa, see David Beach 1980. The Jesuits made converts, including the Mwene Mutapa himself, but Fr Silveira was subsequently killed on charges of witchcraft.

[4] Bourdillon took these estimates from figures of the Catholic Bishops Conference. He noted later 'the number of those who claim affiliation to a church is likely to be much greater than the official estimates of established churches – when I was in the field people often said they were Catholics because their children attended the Catholic school and they attended meetings with priests.' (Bourdillon 2010)

gest a significant degree of underestimation or perhaps the explosive growth of Christian churches since independence in 1980. In either case, although I know of no reliable contemporary figures on church membership (or self-defined Christian identity), it would seem that a majority of Zimbabweans would now categorize themselves as Christians and as followers of particular churches. In addition, active and widespread church-going behaviours are very obvious in both urban and rural settings in Zimbabwe. The matter of allegiance to particular Christian denominations is, within Zimbabwe, partly a consequence of history and geography (or time and place). Early Christian missions in the colonial period (1890 to 1980) were governed by the policy that deliberately sought to control interdenominational rivalry by separating different churches spatially, thus controlling to a large degree the opportunities for cross-proselytizing and subsequent conflict. In this way the scandal of internal Christian division was partly obscured, and yet perpetuated (see Raftopoulos and Mlambo 2009).

A consequence has been that families' church affiliation is often a matter of the area of origin from which they come. Thus, in Manicaland, the Methodists were well established around Old Mutare, the Seventh Day Adventists near Nyazura and the Anglicans dominated between Bonda and St Augustine's in the Penhalonga area. Roman Catholics were widespread but originating in the Triashill mission near Nyanga, and cemented their political prominence through the courageous opposition of Bishop Donal Lamont to state-sanctioned oppression and violence under the Smith regime (1965–1980). These churches also won loyalty through their extensive commitments to community service, particularly in the provision of education and healthcare. In the 1990s approximately 40% of Zimbabwe's education and health service was attributed to the work of churches and their missions. In this decade it has often been said that the only remaining education and health services are those provided through established churches. For example, when the Mutare Hospital was at its lowest ebb, many people made the (relatively) short trip to the Anglican mission hospital near Penhalonga (about 40km).

Nicholas is one of the children from my group. His aunt (his father's sister) is a devout Anglican and gave me this interesting account of the family's religious history:

> Our family came from the Bonda area so we were always Anglicans. That is the way we prayed. When I married it was to a man from Chimanimani and his people were Apostolics. When he got sick he was healed through the prayers of that church so afterwards I too went to the Apostolic church. But my husband was not a churchgoer. After some time I grew tired of going there. I missed my Anglican way. We had our own ways, our own hymns. Now I have gone back and I am at home.

Church membership is a matter of familiar practice and each church offers its own repertoires of hymns, prayers and other forms of worship. Change from one church to another is, however, not unknown or even uncommon. Zionist churches, and more recently charismatic and Pentecostal churches, would appear to have built extensive followings both in urban and rural areas and in opposition to established, mainstream churches. In my experience in Mutare this often leads to an answer, when asked the question 'what church do you belong to?' of 'well, my grandmother's/family's church is [name of mainstream church] but I go to [name of Pentecostal church]'. I have not seen families in conflict over members' decisions to attend different churches from their elders. My observation of young people's church-going habits, however, suggests to me a strong tendency to sample a range of churches. This may relate, in my experience, to the circulation of stories about which church has the most active youth group, or the most compelling preacher, or the greater healing powers. Older, influential family members might see this sampling of a variety of churches as part of the general restlessness of the young. It may not be that such tolerance would extend to longer term commitments as are socially demonstrated in decisions about the right church, for example, in which to celebrate and formalize marriages, or baptize children. I have certainly seen cases of grandparents (mostly grandmothers) insisting on such rites of passage being celebrated in churches seen as those to which the family has been traditionally aligned.

In these ways the social power and reach of churches is an outcome of historical processes as well as the individual commitments of members and the long-term practices of families. The mainstream churches remain influential in their role, and their commitments to social service. Nonetheless, new charismatic and Pentecostal churches are an obvious feature of contemporary Zimbabwe. David Maxwell (2006) has, for example, thoroughly documented the growth of such a church (Zimbabwe Assemblies of God Africa, ZAOGA), which has now reached transnational levels of social penetration and influence. And the explosive growth of charismatic and Pentecostal Christianity has been noted elsewhere in Africa, and across the global South (Robbins 2004, Meyer 1994, 1999, Pfeiffer 2005). ZAOGA is a church which falls within the ambit of the charismatic and Pentecostal; indeed it has its roots in Mutare and Manicaland, and is very popular with young people I know. Charismatic churches in this vein offer their members forms of spiritual fellowship that both penetrate and encompass the social. Thus, for example, such churches operate forms of worship and study that extend well beyond the usual Sunday model of traditional Christianity.

Susan and Priscilla are two girls from our group whose families belong to different churches. (Susan's are Methodists and Priscilla's Apostolic). However, they both go regularly to the ZAOGA church, particularly for weekday 'crusades', while attending their usual churches with their families on Sundays. Susan said:

> ZAOGA has services every night, especially during their outreach crusades, and we like to go to those. There is music and singing which is more modern, and the preachers are younger. They know our ways. Besides we see our friends from school there and if you say,

at home, I am going for the prayer meeting, they will let you go. Going to church is good, everyone knows.

Anthropology and Christianity

There may be some tendency in anthropological perspectives on re-surgent Christianities to over-emphasize the importance of 'lively' forms of worship (and the electric effects of Holy Spirit possession) in drawing and holding large congregations. In a very important work on recent approaches to Christianity within anthropology, a number of scholars point out that extreme diversity characterizes experiences and instantiations of Christianity across the globe. In her incisive introduction, Fenella Cannell writes:

> It may be true, as both Whitehouse and Keane argue here of Protes-tant services they describe, and has also been claimed of mainstream Catholic liturgy, that public worship can at times be mechanical, drained of affect, and can become boring even to its participants. Such routinization may even be a deliberate policy on the part of church leaders, in the interests of member control. But we have also seen that these conformist appearances can be deceptive and that even where they are true, they do not necessarily exclude a deep engagement with questions of Christian faith. (Cannell, 2006: 30)

Detailed observations of both the charismatic and the banal in forms of Christian worship do not, in themselves, account for Christianity's status as 'the success story of globalization' (Robbins 2004) or sub-stantiate an often-assumed relationship between Christian conver-sion and global modernity (Sahlins 1996, Cannell 2006). Neither, as Cannell points out, do older ideas of popular missionary Christianity as exemplars of 'resistance' as, for example, we find in the Comaroffs' (1991) acclaimed account of revivalism amongst Tshidi Methodists in apartheid South Africa. The popular success of missionary Christi-anity amongst colonized peoples cannot only be understood as an example of hybrid resistance and globalized modernity. By way of a contrasting and confounding example, James Fernandez's (1982) extraordinarily detailed account of Fang syncretic Christianity in the Bwiti cult is a compelling picture of a specifically local form of the Christian that is entirely disconnected from wider, global Christian forms or their engagements with modernity. Furthermore, the various commitments of some Christian churches of the global South to deeply conservative social agenda (see Hoad 2007) do not suggest simple relationships between historical experiences of subjugation and current policies of social inclusion or exclusion.

From this brief overview, it should be apparent that it is both impossible and unwise to generalize about Zimbabwean churches or the beliefs and practices of their adherents. Zimbabwean Christianities are urgently in need of detailed study. The purpose of this chapter is to consider diverse churches' roles in mediating children's experiences of living with HIV. The ways in which the churches might understand these mediating roles in terms of their own theologies and pastoral practices can only be gestured towards here.

The sociality of local churches

At ZAOGA's principal Mutare church, for example, worship and the gathering of the congregation for prayer, singing and teaching is very frequently a daily event. Young people I know will attend church every evening and these gatherings have elements that seem to an outsider to supersede the usual understandings of Christian communal worship. Thus, for example, young people will often tell me that they enjoy going to church frequently as it is a place where they meet their friends, enjoy the music and 'learn things'. Such 'things' learnt would seem to include biblical teaching but also economic, and other life-skills. At stake then are also forms of adolescent sociality and education, in addition to spiritual practices. As Maxwell has shown, ZAOGA is one of those churches that have excelled in the development of 'penny capitalism', a phrase that refers to teachings and practices that encourage thrift and joint income-generating projects. Here one is reminded of earlier practices, especially in the Zionist churches, whose communal and active church lives, and care and encouragement for one another's economic well being, generated their reputation for being considerably better off than their (non-Zionist) neighbours. There is ample evidence for such processes in earlier writings on forms of independent African Christianity (see, for example, Bourdillon 1976 and Daneel 1971).

Given the rapid growth and high profile of newer charismatic and Pentecostal churches, however, it is possible to overstate their importance in the overall religious life of many Zimbabweans in Mutare. I have often accompanied children I know in their attendances at a variety of churches and my observation is that all churches, new and old, are extremely well and enthusiastically attended. For example, on any given Sunday the Catholic Cathedral of the Holy Trinity has five masses, all of which are standing-room only. Another interesting tension between common attributions to old and new churches is one I have often heard: old churches are known to be very widely involved in the provision of social, educational and health services. When I asked the carer of one of the children I know whether she received practical help from the charismatic church she said she was a member of, she looked at me with some surprise, saying, 'It's our job to give them money. We're told that the pastor must have new clothes every month.' She clearly did not see the church as a place in which she might find help with food, clothing or the other basic necessities of life. She appeared to understand this is an example of the ways in which worldly greed infiltrated even the church. This provides an interesting contrast with some recent anthropological writing on charismatic Christianity in which a suggestion is made that tithing[5] is seen as deeply empowering in that it permits poor

---

[5] The Christian tithe is the tenth of one's income ritually given to the church, and is practiced in many churches.

members to experience the power of the donor position (Robbins 2004, Bornstein 2006 and Maxwell 2006).

A common feature of social and religious life in Mutare (and elsewhere in Zimbabwe) is religious events called 'crusades'. These are extended events of intensive teaching, proselytization and healing (often held on consecutive evenings over seven or ten days) and are often formed around the visit of a famed preacher (such as the Nigerian head of Christ Embassy, Pastor Chris) and are widely advertised as places in which miracles are sure to occur. 'Come expecting miracles', proclaimed one banner for a famed healer's visit. Many of the children I know, regardless of the churches they usually attend, are keen to attend these events. The reasons for this are many and certainly go beyond the most obvious religious motives. For one thing, these 'crusades' have a carnival atmosphere, often featuring large bands and choirs, and the riveting spectacle of healings (where the healed will often collapse when touched by the healer), and other entertainments such as 'speaking in tongues' and 'the casting out of spirits'. While eager to attend, none of the children I know expect that they themselves will be the recipients of such healing.[6] This is often because they have attended many such events and have never experienced any change in their health. They are, by and large, strict empiricists in these matters and often very witty in their mimicry of particularly pompous or outrageous itinerant preachers.

Giving and getting from the Lord

As we have seen from the history of Christianity in Zimbabwe, the churches have been intensely and centrally involved in the provision of care, health and education to a majority previously largely excluded from such services. Indeed, even after independence in 1980 the established networks of missions across rural areas (where at the

[6] Or, more accurately, they do not articulate such a hope. It may, nonetheless, be a strong, unconscious wish and motivation.

time over 80% of the population still lived) far exceeded sites of worship, but also included hospitals, schools and tertiary training centres, and were integral to the post-colonial government's attempts to expand healthcare and to replace a previous system (geared to the provision of high-quality tertiary care to a very small minority) with a new system in which a bulk of resources would be directed to the primary care of the many. Many missions in rural areas resemble small towns and contain hospitals, schools, and housing for religious and lay staff.

Historians of the Zimbabwean churches (such as Ian Linden, 1979, in relation to the Catholic Church) have carefully documented their commitment to social welfare. The advent of a post-colonial regime which was, at least in its earlier years, committed to social justice and equitable redistribution has now, as we have seen, collapsed into a regime solely concerned with self-aggrandizement, and the pursuit of perpetual, pure power (again see Raftopoulos and Mlambo 2009). As James Ferguson (2006) has pointed out, part of the dynamics at play here can be attributed to the imposition of Structural Adjustment Programmes in the 1990s (as a consequence of the 'triumph' of neo-liberal economics in the West), their catastrophic effects on local economies and political systems, and the ways in which transnational NGOs stepped in as key providers of local political power and economic provision.

Erica Bornstein (2005) has examined the role of World Vision, a Protestant global NGO with extensive commitments in Zimbabwe. In her ethnography, evangelical intensity and the provision of essential services (boreholes, safe drinking water, and nutritional supplements, for example) are intensely imbricated, but also require elaborate performances – of gratitude by the recipients, and of ardent and evangelical enthusiasm by the employees. In a later paper, Bornstein (2006) recounts how the internal performative rituals of the NGO fail in the face of the widening gap between the organization's headquarters in the rich West and its operational sites in spaces of ever deepening poverty (as in Zimbabwe). Again it seems the universality of a monolithic Christianity is at risk of being grossly overstated. We are, perhaps, always more precise to speak of local Christianities. To return to Cannell:

> Christianity is not an arbitrary construct, but it is a historically complex one. It is not impossible to speak meaningfully about Christianity, but it is important to be as specific as possible about what kind of Christianity one means. (Cannell 2006: 7)

Circuits of charity (global and local) undoubtedly sustain many works by Mutare's churches, which in turn sustain their congregations. Nonetheless, in my discussions with young HIV-infected people and their families, such circuits are remote and difficult to comprehend. By contrast they are all aware of local churches as potential sites of immediate help. Thus there is knowledge about which church communities might hand out clothes or food, and on what days, and to which categories of the needy. There is also detailed knowledge about how different churches might choose recipients of their charity. For example, many churches might prioritize the needs of those whom they see as their members.

Many children and carers I know are aware of these categories, and their church-going habits are at least partly formed by the need to remain within the ambit of such categories. To say this, is not, I think, to denigrate their deep spiritual commitments to profound and personal understandings of Jesus and their relationships with churches, singular and plural. Takura's mother explained this to me:

> I could not go on like this if it were not for the Lord Jesus. Every day I pray, and I make my sons pray, even when they want to go outside and play. I say to them we only have food to eat because Jesus has given it to us. We kneel and raise our hands and then we pray like this [demonstrates the Lord's Prayer and the Hail Mary]. We are Methodists in my family but after I married I became a Catholic as that was the church of my husband's family. Every Sunday I take my sons to mass

here [in Dangamvura]. The sisters at the church help us with food, and sometimes with clothing. Now that medicines are hard to find, I know that they give some free medicines at the (named) Church (a Pentecostal and charismatic local church), so we go there too. I am not playing with these churches. Jesus understands.

Everyday theodicies[7]

I receive emails from colleagues and friends in Zimbabwe when I am out of the country. Some end with religious sentiments, and farewells that are religiously inflected. These range from the traditional, 'the peace of Christ be with you', to those that seem stronger and more improvised; 'from the slopes of Calvary' writes one pastor, 'from under the cloud of Satan' sighs another. I mention these as a way to gesture towards the intense religiosity that many Zimbabweans embody and express in their everyday lives. It is a close awareness of the religious as being intensely imbricated in everyday life, and the way in which these imbrications are played out in the most common forms of language. It is also a coded reference to one of the major problems facing resurgent Christian faith in post-colonial Zimbabwe, and that is how to account for the sheer scale and severity of suffering whilst also trying to remain faithful to a belief in a benevolent and all-powerful deity. Theodicy is very much a topical issue.

Churches may be a major site of social growth in contemporary Zimbabwe (and indeed, as I have already outlined, in today's Mutare), but their very popularity requires an answer to the vexing question of how a loving Christian God would allow his faithful people to suffer such extended and severe adversity. This is a question that frequently comes up in my conversations with children and young people who are HIV-positive, frequently ill (and severely so), and cumulatively bereaved. And as the salutations on emails from col-

[7] See footnote 7, p. 11 for a definition of 'theodicy'.

leaugues demonstrate, even Christian leaders (pastors, priests, nuns and the like) perceive their faith in today's Zimbabwe as being one of solidarity with the poor and oppressed, and as requiring convincing explanation of God's willingness to let his people suffer. (This is a generalization and there are notable exceptions). It is a faith that requires a stress on endurance, and an ethos of the long suffering. I have sometimes thought about this as the problem of the theodicy of the ordinary.[8]

One explanation that young people will often give to me about their understanding as to why God would allow them to suffer is that they have failed to demonstrate adequate faith. This seems especially a problem for those who attend, or have strong emotional commitments to, Pentecostal and charismatic churches. One of the more modern developments in such churches, perhaps especially in conditions of poverty or profound economic uncertainty, is that charismatic doctrine popularly referred to as 'the gospel of prosperity' (again see Robbins 2004 and Maxwell 2006) where a central doctrine is that God desires wealth (understood as money, health and possessions of status) for his followers, and will provide it should they demonstrate sufficient faith. The demonstration of faith is here denoted as an absolute trust in the power of God to provide. Such faith is instantiated in giving to the church and its leaders, in the form of tithes, even when one has very little. By a powerful paradox, disdain for the things of this world brings them (the signs and forms of wealth) in abundance for the true believer. For many poor, sick children I know a similar logic often applies to their understanding of their health. Tinashe said to me:

> I know that, if I have faith, God will cure me. This virus will be like a small cold to him. But I have to show this faith. The best way to show that I believe would be to stop these pills. I take pills because I am

8 By 'the theodicy of the ordinary' I refer to the everyday struggles of Christians to make sense of their suffering as opposed to the (more) arcane debates of theologians and academics.

afraid, and I do not have faith. I pray every day that God will help me to find this faith. Then I will stop the pills and God will see my faith and I will be healed. God is waiting to heal me, to bless me, but I am weak.

Many children I know who have struggled with adherence to their medications, have put forward a version of this argument to explain their profound ambivalence to sustaining the regimes of medication. These are ideas about faith, God and the possibilities of healing that they are not alone in. Members of their families and teachers in their churches all propound similar beliefs. It has often seemed to me that the strength of these beliefs, and the behaviours they entail, fluctuate. At times of either greatest health crisis, or of most severe economic strain they would seem to renew their enchanted logic. At any rate, children have constantly returned to these themes, and their seductions, in the conversations with me over the years that I have known them. As we shall see in the ensuing chapter, when death draws near or the capacity to continue to struggle to live wanes (two experiences which may, in the end, amount to much the same thing), this enchanted logic is part of what, paradoxically, allows a withdrawal from treatment and a resignation to death.

Pastors and elders in Pentecostal and charismatic churches often demonstrate a similar ambiguity in relation to spiritual healing, and the products and regimes of medicine. A pastor I know well said to me:

> Yes, these things [medications] can be good. It isn't bad to take them. But why drink water when God is waiting to give you *mahewu* (a nutritious maize-based drink)? We must expect more from God and then he will give it to us.

It seems to me that however subtle the theologies of pastors and other church leaders in relation to these types of statements, the message that children receive is that the use of medications constitutes a failing of faith. Here we have a social collision of considerable importance: the region's greatest health crisis collides with its fastest growing form of religious practice.

The forces of evil

The reverse of the coin of faith is the work of evil. The faithful are not just hobbled by the struggles to achieve requisite levels of faith, and detachment from the false lures of this world, but are also in constant danger from the snares of the forces of evil. In common Christian understanding, evil is represented by the devil. Shona versions of an understanding of evil would, I think, multiply the figures of evil, most obviously to include the horrifying figure of the witch who is a human who indulges in evil for evil's sake (Gelfand 1967, Bourdillon 1976, Colson 2000, Robbins 2004). The witch, however, might well be included in a pantheon of evil that would include other spiritual forces: *ngozi* (aggrieved spirits), *shave* (alien spirits), *nzuzu* (water spirits), and perhaps even all *midzimu* (ancestral spirits).[9] All the children I know believe very strongly in witches (*varoyi*), goblins (*tokoloshi*), water spirits (*nzuzu*) and the like. Evil is ever present and waiting to strike.

Different churches might approach these matters differently, depending on degrees of intellectual sophistication, attempts at enculturation and, possibly, education. Birgit Meyer (1999), examining Pentecostal practice in West Africa, however, suggests most churches in the evangelical/Pentecostal/charismatic spectrum expend considerable energy on casting all non-Christian spiritual belief and practice into the realm of the demonic. Filip de Boeck's accounts of charismatic Christianity and child witches in Kinshasa (2004) demonstrates intense engagements with Pentecostalism and

[9] Again, see Bourdillon 1976, where we see that 'indigenous' forms of Christianity, such as the *vapostori*, explicitly believe in such a pantheon of evil spirits. Indeed, as Robbins (2003) also suggests in relation to the global success of these forms of Christianity, part of the success of Pentecostal and charismatic churches is that they take seriously such spirit beliefs but proclaim The Holy Spirit (of the Christian Trinity) as being more powerful than all other spirit types.

witchcraft eradication of equal intensity and popularity. Robbins (2004) points out that by taking all 'traditional' spiritual forces seriously, charismatic churches greatly enhance their ability to enter into a very wide variety of profoundly various cultural domains while holding their own beliefs and practices relatively stable. Within Zimbabwe, Maxwell, in relation to ZAOGA, also shows extensive church commitment to casting all beliefs in spiritual forms (other than those of the Holy Spirit) into categories of the forbidden and the evil (for the faithful).

In relation, however, to people's everyday practice, it seems to me, matters are somewhat less clear-cut. We have seen how Priscilla's guardians, the Gwaunza family, regard with considerable trepidation how her 'bad luck' (the loss of her parents, the loss of her grandmother, the distance between her and her father's kin, her own ill health) may imply the displeasure of other spirits, specifically an *ngozi*. We have also seen how Mai Takura perseverates on the question of the relationship between her sons and their father's family (including, perhaps, his spirit family, *midzimu*; what Bourdillon refers to as 'spirit elders'). And we shall also see how families burying their dead contrive rituals that span 'traditional' and 'Christian' cosmologies and practices in ways that might seem incommensurate to either traditionalists or Christians.

These personal compromises over matters of spirits, particularly evil spirits such as those represented in the workings of witches, are among the many issues that are not well researched in relation to the various practices of Christianity in Zimbabwe. Lurid tales of the work of witches are staples of Zimbabwean tabloids and, in recent years, have implicated politicians at the highest levels of the state. A few years ago a number of senior cabinet ministers were implicated in paying large sums of public money to a woman, a spirit medium, who was said to be able to produce diesel from rocks.

Paradox in the practice of one church

One church I have come to know well in the course of my fieldwork is one within the mould of charismatic and Pentecostal. As such it is a church where it is said that the gifts of the Holy Spirit (including healing) are available to all. Within such a context of Christian faith where the transcendent is privileged (here I use the distinction between the transcendent and the incarnate that a number of commentators have characterized as one essential oscillation in various forms of Christianity; see Cannell 2006, Keane 2008, Sahlins 1996), there is also committed attention to the material needs of the congregation. The church runs a pharmacy, a school, a feeding scheme and additional services for orphans and widows. The church also has vigorous, elastic and intense engagement with social provision, allowing it to respond rapidly and helpfully to changing (often deteriorating) conditions in Mutare.

These activities would be less unusual in a more mainstream church where principles of service, especially to the poor, are integral to official teaching. And indeed, in my conversations with leaders in this church, there certainly are clear commitments to providing for the needy. However, interestingly, in conversations with young people who attend some services at this church, there is a great deal more confusion. Such confusion seems especially complex in relation to the church's pharmacy and drug supply service. Kuda said to me:

> But they teach here that prayer is enough. I don't understand why they are giving pills. Is it to see who has faith and who does not?

Furthermore, I know of no church in Mutare, mainstream or new, which pays serious attention to the educational needs of young people in relation to emergent sexualities and reproductive health. All churches, it would seem, teach stern versions of abstinence and none counsel the use of condoms. When I asked one church elder, who is also a doctor, whether he thought such teachings problematic, he said:

> Abstinence is the Lord's way. If I know of a young couple who are in a committed relationship I might privately counsel the use of condoms but no true church leader could do so openly. Even though we all know that children are sexually active at young ages. Abstinence is the teaching of the Scriptures.

Isolation and the faithful

Given that most of the children I know, and their families, are regular attenders at church, and devout believers in various forms of Christianity, and given too that such a high proportion of Zimbabweans have had some close, intimate relationship with HIV, it is remarkable that none of the children I know well ever speak of their illnesses in church contexts. For example, Priscilla tells me that she 'prays in her heart' at church about her many worries about her health and her future, but cannot conceive of a situation in which she might think it helpful to speak openly or to directly elicit the care and attention of her fellow congregants (quite a number of whom must be in the same situation as her). Indeed most of the children tell me that their fellow Christians would not be any more open or tolerant, and that, in effect, the risks of stigma and devastating exposure would be just as great. A number of children have told me that, were one to speak about one's struggles with HIV in church, the information would quickly travel outside the church and all confidentiality would be lost.

Children do not recount these circumstances without emotion. Many tell me that they would find the greatest comfort in being able to share their struggles and fears with their fellow worshippers. It seems to me that they interpret this 'failure', not as an indictment of Jesus or of Christianity, but purely of their fellow believers. Consider the following incident:

A Sunday mass in the Catholic Church in Dangamvura. The building is packed. The congregation is segregated by gender; men to one side, women to the other. There appear to me to be equal numbers of both. The music is haunting. The Kyrie in particular moves me to tears. I see Tinashe near the back. He has been suffering for some months now from a terrible skin rash and his right eye is swollen shut. His clothes are ragged. I can't see his mother. He doesn't take communion. Afterwards I see him again in the crowd outside. He stands alone. As I edge towards him through the crowd, I see a small girl (perhaps 5 or 6) offer him her handkerchief? Her mother looks down and sees Tinashe. She snatches the cloth from her daughter. From her bag she produces instead a paper tissue. She offers it to Tinashe. His eye is weeping now. He reaches out to take it and, a fraction of a second before he grasps it, she lets go. The tissue falls to the ground. The small girl goes to pick it up. Her mother pulls her away and scolds her. Tinashe remains motionless, his eyes on the ground. (Fieldnotes)

This is not offered as an indictment of indifference in a Catholic community. I could find such examples from church services in all of the possible range of alternatives. It does suggest the simple but profoundly painful slights that the obviously ill and poor are subject to.

Of course, there are some exceptions. Kuda is now a 20-year-old girl. She lives with her mother's sister, and has done so for as long as she can remember. She is also one of the healthiest children I know. She has suffered from comparatively few opportunistic infections, is not stunted and shows no other obvious forms of illness. In fact she is a tall, attractive and healthy looking young woman. Her family are devout Anglicans, but she herself has been attending Christ Embassy for about two years now. (Christ Embassy is a Pentecostal/charismatic church, originating in Nigeria and now very popular in Zimbabwe). About a year ago, Kuda told me that she had decided to tell her congregation that she was HIV-positive. She told me that she thought that this would make her 'feel more free'. I was concerned lest she expose herself to abuse. Kuda, however, went ahead with her act of 'coming out'. The other children were very intrigued with this and often asked Kuda about her experience. She reported that she had not suffered any isolation in the church and had, in fact, received praise and encouragement for her bravery and suffering. However, after some months, Kuda was feeling less sanguine about her experience. She told me that she was feeling that her fellow Christians were less sympathetic to her, and 'don't like me to talk to their children'. She felt a growing sense of isolation.

> At first I was praised. 'You are so brave,' they said. Everyone was applauding me. I felt so good. I had worried about doing this thing before but afterwards I said to myself, 'Ah, but God has guided me to do the right thing'. I thought I would have strong friendships but now I see that people are afraid. What do they say at home? I stand alone sometimes.

The sense of being intensely isolated as someone who is HIV-positive within one's community of believers appears to be common to young people who attend a variety of churches. I have not heard of any churches or religious communities who have tried or managed to create the possibility for openness with safety for its members who are HIV-positive.

Sincerity and comfort

It seems to me that the most immanent and immediate form of Christian practice for the children and their families who I know in Mutare, occurs in the realm of the domestic. It is in the spaces and practices of private family prayer, and other devotional practices (particularly the reading and recitation of sacred, biblical texts such as the Psalms), that the people I know understand their beliefs to be crucial to their lives regardless of their institutional commitments

over time to one or another church. By my use of the word 'immanent' here I refer both to the lived instantiations of faith in everyday
life as well as their relationship to a living Jesus, the immanent God
central to Christian doctrine.

Clearly such personal devotional practice is developed and sustained within the context of relationships with spiritual teachers,
both within families (for example, elders such as grandmothers who
are seen as living lives of particular spiritual intensity and significance) and within churches, with inspirational preachers (or not),
other worshippers and a living-out of values and practices seen as
deeply imbued with the teachings of the Christian Gospels. The
relationships between personal belief and practice, and the practices
and beliefs within specific churches are obviously closely related and
intertwined, but are also not isomorphic. As Webb Keane (2007)
has demonstrated, these interactive relationships are crucial to the
development of the modern, sincere subject:

> First, sincerity is a metadiscursive term. It characterizes a relationship
> between words and interior states. To be sincere is to utter words that
> can be taken to be isomorphic with beliefs or intentions. As a meta-
> discursive term, then, sincerity is a component of linguistic ideology.
> It posits a relationship between speech and its imputed sources in the
> speaker's self: sincere speech makes that interior state transparent.
> It adds and subtracts nothing in words that was not already there in
> thought. (Webb Keane, 2007: 316)

For Keane, this ardent search for pure belief and its exact transcrip-
tion in sincere speech leads to 'an anxious transcendence'. The attempt to reach a transcendent (indeed, somewhat obscure) God is a
matter for daily reapplication, and the weathering of a no less continual uncertainty.

Amongst the children I know, and their families, belief and devotional practice are daily instantiated. Such instantiation takes the
forms of devotional practices (daily prayer ranging from recitation

to spontaneity), close relationships with sacred texts (in vernacular translation), and a striving to act in ways believed to be resonant with Gospel values (such as hospitality and charity even when there is very little to share). These are all attempts to create and sustain spiritual sincerity.

Furthermore, it would seem to me that one goal and outcome of a commitment to spiritual sincerity is profound comfort. Amidst circumstances of the direst suffering, many children and young people, and their families and networks, find their greatest comfort in their sense of close and intense relationships with a loving God, and an ever-present Jesus. As Ramie Targoff (2001) has shown in relation to the development of forms of popular devotional practice (particularly, prayer) in early modern England, people develop intense emotional attachments to sacred and devotional texts. Such attachments may be said to supersede the theological meanings actually inhering in such texts, and certainly they appear to exceed intellectual, theological work on their significance. We will see in the next chapter how, in the course of a lonely and painful death, one boy I know found great comfort in a repeated reading of Psalm 23. So great was the comfort he obtained from this, that, in a letter to me written shortly before his death, he urges a reading of the same text on me, apparently convinced that the words, imbued with his fervour (imbued indeed with the fervour of all the faithful), might bring comfort to me too.

Summary

'The body, then, has had to bear the structures of society in a particularly intense and notably painful way.' Marshall Sahlins (1996: 415) remarks on the vicissitudes of the body in relation to society and, in particular, the imbrications of religion and society as embodied, in his remarkable paper, 'The Sadness of Sweetness', originally delivered as a Sidney Mintz Lecture. His paper seeks to delineate the ways in which Christian cosmology and anthropology have long had a close though largely concealed relationship. Fenella Cannell (2006), in her re-examination of an anthropology of Christianity, refers to Christian belief as 'the return of anthropology's repressed', and as its 'repugnant social other'.

The resurgence of various forms of Christianity across the globe certainly requires of anthropology a new engagement with forms of religious belief which it had, perhaps, long thought rather too obvious and close to the western disciplinary 'home' for serious study. In contemporary Africa the power and rapid growth of African Christianity, in a bewildering variety of forms, calls for a great deal more serious study. In Mutare, in eastern Zimbabwe, the lives of children infected with HIV are closely mediated by their involvement in a range of churches, and imbued with both meaning and practical significance through the beliefs and practices of Christians, others, and their own.

Christianity, and its instantiations in particular churches, theologies and devotional practices, is not the only form of spiritual understanding available to children growing up HIV-positive in Mutare, although it is undoubtedly now the most important. Older cosmologies of 'traditional' Shona religion persist alongside Christianities. The palpable evil of the world is still explained with recourse to the figure of the witch, the spirits (of ancestors, aliens and water) and a range of other clan and totem taboos. Nor is it only persistent evil that is explained through the tropes of the 'traditional'. Bad luck, ill health and poor fortune all can and do find plausible explanations in these domains. Again we might reflect on Richard Werbner's (1997) insightful account of the Christian and modern/ traditional and primitive binary that obscures so much in this field.

It does seem to me though that many of the children I know, along with their families, struggle principally to make themselves into good Christians, to become 'sinners deserving of redemption', in Joel Robbins' account of Christian conversion in Papua New Guinea

(2004), and to be the 'sincere subjects' of Webb Keane's Indonesian converts (2007). Christianity, a moving and fabulously varied object, remains the piercing sweetness to be sought for, and held to, against all odds.

6

One day this will all be over
Dying, death and grief

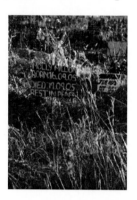

Introduction

The ethnography up to this point has looked at many aspects of the lives of children growing up HIV-positive in Mutare. I have considered the locale and forms of the study; and the place of these children within their families and kin groups and the nature of the care they receive there. I have also have examined the forms their illnesses take and the mediating power of institutions, primarily hospitals and churches, which give shape to their lives and their experiences of illness. Beyond all these important elements in their lives, however, hangs the impenetrable, unpredictable and opaque reality of death. The children encounter death daily through their multiple experiences of bereavement, and through their knowledge of their own possible, though unpredictable, deaths.

How shall we speak of death and of dying in an anthropological register? Writing in the *Annual Reviews of Anthropology* in 1984, Phyllis Palgi and Henry Abramovitch noted:

> When reading through the anthropological literature in one large sweep, one is left with the impression of coolness and remoteness.

The focus is on the bereaved and the corpse but never on the dying. (1984: 385)

Reading Michael Bourdillon, the last anthropologist to attempt a grand narrative of the Shona peoples, as we have done throughout, this observation might be borne out. Although he devotes an entire chapter to death and its social consequences (the rituals of grieving, burial and 'bringing the spirit home'), the tone is one of objective distance. It seems that the elision of the emotions that accompany an unnatural, premature death, a form perhaps of 'matter out of place' as Mary Douglas (1966) remarked of pollution,[1] is fully accomplished. In a passage that will become instructive later on, Bourdillon has this to say:

> A person who has acquired full adult status requires more cooling ritual than a person who died without progeny, indicating the former is believed to be more dangerous. At the funeral of a very small child, the danger is considered to be so slight that some attendants do not bother to purify themselves after it.[2] (Bourdillon 1976: 205)

It should perhaps be noted, as Palgi and Abramovitch do, that it has rarely been an aim of anthropology to attend to the emotions of death. The more general aim has been to consider the social structures and processes that accompany it and that guide the bereaved through their loss as a form of extreme liminality, on the one hand, and potential pollution, on the other. However there has been at least one remarkable exception to this general rule, although it is not mentioned in the Palgi and Abramovitch review. In 1978, Myra Bluebond-Langner published *The Private Worlds of Dying Children*,

---

[1] The phrase originated from William James, but was made common currency by Douglas.
[2] 'Most people, however, maintain that such an omission is wrong: as one old man put it, "A dead child is a person of God (*munhu waMwari*): we clap hands to him (the spirit of the child, before leaving the grave)." Even the weakest of spirits is feared and must be treated with respect.' (Bourdillon 1976: 205)

an ethnography of a children's cancer ward in a large American hospital. Here the dying of children is foregrounded and we are given a vivid picture of children, often very young, who are aware of their own impending deaths and yet whose major preoccupation appears to be one of protecting their parents from this knowledge. I think it is a remarkable work but one, however, with limited application to our concerns here. The deaths described by Bluebond-Langner are exceptional, untimely and intensely mediated by the institution (in this case the hospital). The dying and dead children I wish to consider here are only too unexceptional and, as we have seen, there are few institutions in contemporary Zimbabwe able to mediate their deaths. In my use of the word 'unexceptional' here I refer to the wholesale nature of death in contemporary Zimbabwe (some estimates suggest that there are more than 3,000 HIV-related deaths a week). Of course, for the loved ones of those who have died, death is always exceptional.

Nancy Scheper-Hughes' *Death without weeping: the violence of everyday life in Brazil* (1992) is another ethnography with particular reference to our subject here. Her concern is to document the lives of shanty dwellers in one of Brazil's poorest areas. In particular she is concerned to understand the lives of poor women who have lost many babies at, or shortly after, birth. These are multiple losses under conditions of extreme hardship: poverty, hunger, political oppression. (And thus much like circumstances in contemporary Zimbabwe). She is bewildered to find an absence of mourning, even a withdrawal from the care of infants who appear unlikely to survive by their mothers. While I find her work speaks to much of the everyday extremity faced by people in Zimbabwe, I have not found an absence of mourning or a deliberate withdrawal from care. I have found an exhaustion with care and loss, but I do not think these are the same things. In her introduction she has this to say, which may form a pertinent opening to our thinking here:

The act of witnessing is what lends our work its moral (at times its almost theological) character. So-called participant observation has a way of drawing the ethnographer into spaces of human life where she or he might really prefer not to go at all and once there doesn't know how to go about getting out except through writing, which draws others there as well, making them party to the act of witnessing. (Scheper-Hughes 1992: 7)[3]

Local prognosis

In the West in the late 1980s and early 1990s, HIV infection equated with certain death, within a relatively short time span. The advent of antiretroviral drugs in the late 1990s brought with it, again in the West, a profound shift (in the imaginary temporality) from certain death to chronic, manageable illness. There has perhaps been an idea that this shift has accompanied antiretroviral drugs into poorer countries, and therefore that HIV has become, potentially at least, universally a chronic disease. One of my more important and authoritative informants, a local paediatrician, remarked to me:

I mentioned to a colleague of mine at (a well-known British children's hospital) that HIV in children could now be considered to have a prognosis similar to many forms of diabetes, that is, with appropriate care a patient might expect to lead a relatively normal life into their sixties. He said that he had also made this assumption but that, on reviewing the literature and his own clinical experience, and given the parlous state of many healthcare systems, he had come to the conclusion that the more appropriate parallel was to an illness such as cystic fibrosis (a much more severe illness affecting children who rarely live past their twenties).

---

[3] The topic of witnessing has become an important one in contemporary social anthropology, where the anthropologist is also seen as 'a witness'. See George Marcus (2010) for such an argument in relation to the role of the anthropologist in conflict and post-conflict societies.

This is a remarkable statement and expresses a point of view that I do not think is widely known outside of highly professionalized circles.[4] Certainly I have never heard reference to this rather stark version of HIV-related prognosis (with ARV treatment) amongst children and their caregivers in conversations I have had in Zimbabwe. Recently I happened to be present at a meeting between Priscilla and her doctor (the same doctor whose conversation with me I have reported here). He was generally pleased with her progress, her (marginal) weight gain and her treatment compliance. She hesitated. She had an urgent question she wished to ask the doctor. No, she did not want me to leave the room. She began by relating an incident from home in which her cousins had been sitting with the adults and discussing their ambitions for the future: what jobs they might get, whether they would want to be married and how many children they would like. 'I just kept quiet,' she said, 'I didn't know if I had a future.' Now she was crying. 'How long will it be before I die?' The doctor tried valiantly to comfort her with an account of current research on life expectancy among those on ARVs (but an account, however, considerably more vague than that I have reported above). Observing their conversation, it seemed to me that it was not the answer that Priscilla was seeking, or needing. Any answer was perhaps beside the point. Despite her youth, Priscilla knows about unpredictability and uncertainty, and she certainly knows about death.

Ambivalent lives

Priscilla is one of the children whom I have come to know well during the course of my fieldwork and about whom I have had much to say in previous chapters. To briefly recap, her father died when she was an infant and she has no memories of him although she knows that her parents were estranged and in dispute over mainte-

[4] However, see Lopman et al. (2007) for a recent view confirming this from public health research in Zimbabwe.

nance payments. Her mother died when she was about nine. She had lived with her mother and her grandmother (her mother's mother), and when her mother died she continued to live with her grandmother, with whom she was very close and who seems to have played a crucial role in mediating the loss of her mother. Her grandmother was very close to Priscilla until her own death of cancer. Priscilla speaks of her dreams of both her mother and grandmother: 'they smile at me, my mother smiles, and my grandmother tells me to be good and laughs.' This is comforting, but she also identifies 'home' as being where they are. When she feels most dislocated and alone, it is the sense of loved ones waiting for her in heaven (*padenga* being the Shona word in question and literally meaning *above*) that she is homesick for.

As we have seen from our previous encounter with Priscilla and her family, she is a young woman (who looks like a girl) with a profound ambivalence towards her life, filled as it is with struggle, constraint and deprivation. I have frequently heard from her the phrase, 'this life is too hard for me'. As we have seen, her ambivalence about her life has had repeated and severe impact on her adherence to treatment regimes. We might say that she is only loosely and intermittently attached to life. Death has a seductive hold on her, appearing to promise peace, reunion with loved ones and a cessation of struggle. How might we understand this ambivalent attitude to life? In other places (such as western clinics) I think there would be immediate recourse to the languages of mental health, specifically of depression and other related mood disorders. Priscilla would be understood, and treated, as demonstrating some form of co-morbidity (HIV plus depression). Her ambivalent attachment to life, and its expression in her uncertain adherence to treatment, would be understood as a form of the incomprehensible, a form that is of mental illness.[5] The

---

[5] João Biehl (2005) uses his work with a single woman in a Brazilian hospice/shelter to demonstrate a similar form of a way of living with illness, which is 'incomprehensible' to her medical carers.

clinic in Mutare that I have investigated, as noted before, does not have mental health professionals or even anti-depressants. Is this then only a case of a lack, an absence of appropriate treatments as a consequence of poverty and a failed health system, or are there other elements that might allow us a more nuanced understanding of the issues and impulses at stake here?

Consider the death of another child of my acquaintance, Stephen. He was one of the first children referred to the group. He lived with his grandmother (mother's mother) as both his parents were dead. He was about 14 years old at the time, and was perhaps the most obviously psychologically distressed of the initial group. He had developed an eccentric, although demonstrative, habit of covering his ears with his hands whenever conversations about his illness arose. Early on in the development of the group, perhaps its third meeting, he had not arrived on time. His grandmother entered the room unannounced some 20 minutes after we had begun. I looked up expecting Stephen to follow after her in his usual somewhat reluctant way. 'Oh,' I said, slightly annoyed at their lateness but hoping that I merely looked welcoming, and looking past her for Stephen, 'Hullo, welcome, where is Stephen?' There was a short pause during which I noticed that his grandmother looked quite dazed, and she said, 'I'm sorry. I came to tell you that Stephen is dead,' and burst into tears.

It seemed to me that the silence in the room was suddenly very alert as I hastily rose to attempt to comfort Stephen's grandmother. He had died after an acute bout of malaria, probably worsened by his weakened immune system, and, said his grandmother, 'in great fear and distress'. In the wake of the event, the rest of the children showed sorrow, distress and fear, but were also strangely emboldened to speak, for the first time with me, of their own experiences of deaths, and funerals, and the strange relief that can sometimes be brought by various forms of grief. 'It's good,' said one, 'that we can cry for him, and that he doesn't have to listen anymore.' As they spoke they acknowledged a relief that it had not been one of them who had died, and a fear that they might be next, that death could come swiftly and unannounced. In this conversation grief and the fear of death came palpably into the room, not as something strange, but as something that they were all aware of but deeply unaccustomed to speaking of or acknowledging in any way.

The consolations of psychology revisited

So what shall we do with these mundane, banal though fiercely painful emotions? How shall we understand the grief and fear of children facing their own deaths while living in the aftermath of the deaths of their loved ones? High modernity in critical social theory offers us the distinctions of Deleuzian affect[6] which I fear comes close to a very impoverished account of human emotion, and biomedicine/ neuroscience offers us the treatable versions of mood disorders.[7] I am unconvinced by either, since it seems to me that both suggest an avoidance of the pain and, in this sense, suggest forms of hope (inscribed variously on the social or the physical bodies). In either case hard social realities are elided. I am not alone in the concern that anthropology might offer a fuller account of human life and death than either of these theoretical domains have managed so far. João Biehl, Arthur Kleinman and Byron Good call for us to go 'beyond formulations of human nature that rely on neurobiology and biologically based theories of psychopathology, now dominant.' (2007: 16). I want to urge an ethnography of those offering the least scope for

[6]   In Deleuzian thought, affect is not personal. He and Guattari (his frequent co-worker) distinguish between feeling (personal and biographical), emotion (social) and affect (prepersonal). Gilles Deleuze was a highly influential figure in late twentieth century French philosophy. The work on the meanings of affect appears primarily in their magnum opus, *A Thousand Plateaus: Capitalism and Schizophrenia*.

[7]   In western biomedicine, mood disorders cover forms of depression and anxiety, and are widely treated with medications and/or forms of psychotherapy.

the application of an opiate of hope:[8] HIV-positive, poor children living precariously in a failing state; an aesthetic by contrast of grief and resignation whose only usefulness might lie in the attempt at fulsome witness.

The stoicism of the stance I receive in large part from Sigmund Freud's 'disillusionment' (as taken from his sombre 1915 essay *Thoughts for the Times on War and Death*'[9] written in the wake of his own eldest son's death in the Great War' and recalling his bleak dictum that psychoanalysis could only ever offer, at its best, a move from 'neurotic misery to general unhappiness'), as well as from the social distaste of Henry David Thoreau (1854) (for, surely, the recluse of Walden is nothing if not weary of his fellow humans and their constant strivings). The challenge is offered in these tales drawn from my ethnography. I wonder what emerges when I (the anthropologist at home, or at least hybridly so) then allow myself to mourn the end of hope, as especially personified and animated in the deaths and dying of these children now so well known to me as to be my own; and the apparent indifference of other realms and beings to our several plights?

This might be an opportune moment, then, to consider the usefulness of Freud's influential theory of grief as offered in *Mourning and Melancholia* (1917), where the former is taken as 'successful' grief and the latter as a 'failure'. Once again it seems to me that Freud's work here is based on death as exceptional, in the sense that we might all

---

[8]   From this it will be clear to the reader that I have come to hold a view of 'hope' that is deeply critical, less than optimistic, and certainly not in keeping with Christian notions of 'hope' as a cardinal virtue. It seems to me that hope is best understood as a form of protective denial against unbearable emotional pain, *pace* Freud.

[9]   'We may draw one consolation from our reflections so far: that our injury and painful disillusion at the uncivilized behaviour of our fellow citizens of the world in this war were unjustified. They were based upon an illusion to which we had yielded. Those citizens, in fact, have not fallen as far as we feared, because they had not risen nearly so far as we had imagined.' (Freud 1915)

find the death of a close loved one as being an event of some impact. I do not think that it is a theory constructed to account for mass death and cumulative bereavement. We would need to rethink his terms for such a situation. In this regard it would seem to me that 'normal grieving' (a strange oxymoron at any time) is beyond reach, and necessarily so in abnormal conditions. In the latter, melancholia would logically seem the healthier endpoint.[10]

Later theorists of death, dying and grief (Kübler-Ross 1969, Lindemann 1979) furthered Freud's work with more detailed accounts of grief and mourning, with rigorous attempts to understand the processes as exceptional experience that yet remained within normal parameters. Once again, however, they are not theories intended to explain mass death and cumulative bereavement. There are no theories of death and grief that do so. The closest we may come is through the stark Holocaust memoirs of Primo Levi (1959, 1965, 1988), or Robert Jay Lifton's (1987) attempts to understand the catastrophic consequences of mass death in Hiroshima and Nagasaki. We have yet to begin to imagine even the outlines of a theory of grief to account for loss, and its social and personal expressions, in the wake of such appalling suffering.

Languages of death

Let us turn to the end of yet another child. Persistence is HIV-positive, poor, weakening and precariously socially linked. A 14-year-old boy, he lives with his mother and his father's family. His father is dead. His mother's position amongst paternal kin is tenuous and disputed. Marriage negotiations were never concluded and bride wealth never fully paid. On my return from a period in the United States he was absent from group meetings and said by the other children

---

[10] Freud's writing and theories are considerably more subtle and sophisticated than my brief summary here. I urge the reader to read Freud's own work on the subject to see whether they agree with my (brutally) short summary here.

to have 'lost hope' (*ha'atarisa*/lit: he cannot see forward). In the family's urban home (which I visited in an attempt to track him down) the wife of his father's brother (*tete waPersistence*), offered an account of how he had been abducted by *nzuzu* (water spirits). This account was offered spontaneously in response to my attempts to ask where he was and what the other children had meant by referring to him as having 'lost hope':

> Persistence is not here. He was walking in the forest when he came to a pool. He was taken by the water spirits who are known to live there. We do not know what will happen. We are waiting. We may not grieve for someone taken by a water spirit, he will not come back.[11]

She offered an elaborate account of the water spirit world in response to my perplexity. *Nzuzu* are water spirits who live beneath water, she told me, in worlds closely approximating aspects of our own: inter alia, they are white, have long hair, live in cities and towns, have factories, houses and livestock and eat fish and mud. While accounts of water spirits abound in the southern African ethnographic record, I have not seen any of such specificity or such resonance with regard to a diminishing modernity, indicating that they may be specific to, and recently embellished by, urban Manyika people. Elements of reference to an otherwise remote, receding and inaccessible modernity appear to be evident here, recalling, amongst others, Filip De Boeck's accounts of the macabre modernities of child witches in Kinshasa (2004), as well as James Ferguson's (1999) 'anthropology of decline' in the (previously wealthy) urban and peri-urban spaces of the Zambian copperbelt.

The fullest ethnographic account of the water spirits in Shona thought and belief is to be found in the work of Herbert Aschwanden (1989), who collected myths in the 1960s and 1970s amongst

---

[11] This is my rough translation. The last sentence is almost an exact translation of an avoidance rule (a form of proverbial wisdom often taught to children in the form of simple rhyming couplets) given by Michael Gelfand (1979: 147) as *kuchema munhu atorwa nenzuzu.*

rural Karanga people (a Shona sub-group, whose lands lie south-west of Mutare). In the Karanga sub-dialect water spirits are known as *njuzu*, as opposed to the Manyika version of *nzuzu* (the people of Mutare are primarily Manyika). For Aschwanden's informants, the pool (a permanent source of water which persists even through the driest seasons) is always a sacred space, and its guardians are the *njuzu*. Aschwanden gives this account of the origins of the *njuzu* from one of his oldest informants:

> God created human beings, and they were all good. Then God thought that there were too many of them, and he divided them into two groups. He said to one group: 'go into the opening of this moun-tain which I have made for you'. The people went in, with their women and their cattle. Thus the '*vari pasi*' (those below) came into being .... These creatures below ground are ... beings like humans; only after death do they attain a spirit nature too. They experience their sub-terranean world as we humans do ours, and a blue sky spans both worlds. They also build huts, and have cattle and fields. (Aschwanden 1989: 187-8)[12]

We might usefully begin here by noting the similarities between this account from a rural informant collected over 50 years ago, and the 'modernized' version that *tete wa*Persistence offered me (huts, fields and cattle have become houses, factories and white people). Humans are abducted for unknown reasons but are generally lost thereafter. Other informants tell me that *nzuzu* 'trick' abductees into eating their food. Consumption then marks a point of the irrevers-ible. Return thereafter is impossible. Abductees are sometimes said to have then become the servants of the spirits. Abduction does not equate with physical death. The rituals of a death are not followed. Notably temporalities are altered. The length of time of an abduction

---

[12] Note that the *vari pasi* (those who live below and of whom *njuzu* form a sub-group are but one of three groups of humans which also includes ourselves and the *vari padenga* those above).

is not a human temporality. *Nzuzu* are said to have their own time.

Two exceptions remain: the abductee is returned with the potential for healing powers, or the spirits (who listen for sounds of grieving at abductees' homesteads) are convinced that the abductee is not mourned and is therefore returned. Here, in an intriguing paradox, the crucial factor is the absence of audible mourning. The abductee who is unmourned is not valued by the *nzuzu* and thus might be returned. *Tete wa*Persistence offered this as an explanation for the absence of mourning in the homestead for the 'disappearance' of the child. Public mourning would endanger the child further. The emotion with which she told me this tale, however, was one marked by anxiety, fear and restrained grief.

The paternal family are also members of an indigenous apostolic (and syncretic) sect, which originated in the 1940s from more immediate followers of Johannes Marange.[13] Here a discourse of charismatic, socially conservative, indigenously nuanced Christianity does not, however, enter into an outright, predictable conflict with the tale of the *nzuzu*. On the contrary, the two tales are intertwined and commodious of paradoxical spiritual belief. The spirits are undoubtedly emotionally indifferent to the overwhelming daily realities of Persistence and his family. They are not compassionate. Their interventions into the life of Persistence and his family are neither benign nor malign. They are both uncanny and inscrutable.

Frankly, I do not know what to make of the *tete*'s account of *nzuzu*, especially when we compare it to the later account of what happened to Persistence, as we shall see. I later discovered that this woman and her sister are the sole survivors in Persistence's father's family. Everyone else has died. I had thought the homestead was very quiet but as it was a weekday I had assumed that other members were out on business or errands. I have wondered whether what she was saying was also a way of telling me something about that home as being a

---

[13] Apostles/*vapostori*: see Bourdillon (1991: 297) for a fuller account, and also Daneel (1971).

site of death, and the absence of mourning as explicable as a certain waiting and a form of exhaustion. These are only speculations.

Members of Persistence's family in town (*mhuri wataundi*) had told me that Persistence had returned with his mother to his grandmother's (his mother's mother) rural homestead (*kumusha*), and that it was in this place that he had been abducted. The homestead is in the Makoni district of Manyika, some 100kms west of Mutare, near the town of Rusape. This is an area that is highly volatile and the scene of intense political violence. It is the personal fiefdom of a ZANU-PF cabinet minister and local warlord, famous for his public remark that he would prefer to see Zimbabwe lose three-quarters of its population as they were not 'true revolutionaries'. An area then where life is marked politically as indifferent, dispensable, irrelevant (if not actively anathema) to resurgent nationalist revolution and anti-(neo) colonial struggle.

Persistence's end

Some six months after my return, Persistence's mother unexpectedly appeared at one of our Friday afternoon meetings. She had come to tell me that Persistence had died some six months previously. She did not dispute the *tete's* account of abduction by *nzuzu*, nor did she seem surprised by it. She did not, in fact, engage with the story at all. Her account was in a different register (perhaps one assumed to be more palatable to western, medical and Christian ears):

> In late November 2007, Persistence fell ill. He was admitted to hospital. The diagnosis was of probable malaria. The symptoms were high fever, delirium and malaise. He did not respond to medication. He lost time. He cried. He cried to me to take him *kumusha*. So I took him although the nurses told me to stay. I could not see him cry. When we first arrived home he was stronger but then he slowly grew worse again. He lay down all day. He would cry to me. He became like a small child again (*mwana mudiki*). I would put him on my back. He

would quieten a while. He would say 'come *amai* (mother) let us pray', or he would wake me at night and say '*Amai* let us read the Bible'. He could not eat. Everything he ate, he vomited. I had no money for good food. One day he cried loudly and then was still. I did not know what to do. I put him on my back like a baby (*wambereki*) and sang to him of Jesus. His grandmother came and said 'he is dead (*akafa*)'. I was lost for a long time. He wrote you a letter on the last day but until now I was unable to come here.

The letter was a small sheet of newsprint, stapled together and addressed to me in Persistence's handwriting. It read (in English):

My loving father. I have struggled a long time. I have tried. I am very sick. Read Psalm 23. Remember my mother's family. Your loving son.

I wept.

Later I re-read the psalm which I knew well since it is a favourite of Christian piety and a standard of Christian burials. I reproduce it here:

Psalm 23:
1   The Lord is my shepherd, I shall not want./
2   He makes me lie down in green pastures, he leads me beside quiet waters,/
3   he restores my soul. He guides me in paths of righteousness for his name's sake. /
4   Even though I walk through the valley of the shadow of death, I will fear no evil, for you are with me; your rod and your staff, they comfort me./
5   You prepare a table before me / in the presence of my enemies. / You anoint my head with oil; /my cup overflows. /
6   Surely goodness and love will follow me / all the days of my life,/ and I will dwell in the house of the Lord forever. (New International Version)

In my shocked grief, at first, this read as a cliché, and my failure to be comforted distressed me further, marking greater distance between me and my 'loving son'. Over time though, thinking of my child's deathbed message to me, I too have been comforted by this text. Such sacred texts carry profound emotional associations, reinforced by repetition over lives, polished by use, which may well supersede their specific meanings, theological weight or identification with their origins (see Targoff 2001). Thereafter, it seems to me, we might also wonder about the way in which the repetition of sacred text or prayer may well provide words at moments when the horror of life threatens to render all experience unspeakable.

His mother was further distressed as she had had no money for a 'proper burial': no coffin, no cement, and no headstone. We were both temporarily comforted by my promise that I would find money for the headstone. In such small ways does an activism and a philanthropy distract us from our unbearable loss, our pernicious grief. I do not think she was entirely motivated by a desire for financial help, as she did not immediately return to claim the money. I would have felt much better had she done so and had I had the chance to display my usefulness, my indispensable western power of wealth. Instead I remained with this note and its overwhelming incorporation of me into a world of loving kin, so different from the realities. Persistence had offered me a salve of being, of continued usefulness to his family. It is a usefulness I greatly wish I could have exercised. I too have found myself lost in time.

Despair and resignation

There is a sense in which I find it useful to think of these differing accounts as idioms of despair and resignation. Priscilla longs to be with the peaceful dead who loved her, Stephen passes through great fear to a place where he will be spared future listening, and Persistence is variously abducted by uncanny water spirits or becomes one of the well-cared-for flock of the 'good Shepherd'.[14]

[14] For Christians, 'the good shepherd' is a reference (indeed, an honorific title) for Jesus, who himself appears to have used such metaphors in his teachings.

Another child I knew, Nicholas, in his long, last illness (in which he too, with the active connivance of his family, refused treatment) always spoke to me, with considerable humour, about 'being in the waiting room of death' and of 'being next in the queue' (a particularly mordant witticism coming from a Zimbabwean well accustomed to lengthy queues and interminable waiting). I was greatly distressed by Nicholas's refusal of treatment and I spent quite some time talking to his family and trying to argue that they should take him to the hospital. They always politely listened to me, agreed and then, when I had left, carried on as before. They had taken him to his rural home as well, which was in a small farming area quite close to the town. His father's sister became one of my closest informants and a good friend.

She herself, a devout Christian, was critical of her brother's family's care of this boy. On her weekends, when she was not working, she would go to the homestead and spend the day both caring for Nicholas and remonstrating with other family members. He had been moved to a separate sleeping hut, ostensibly to spare him noise and bustle. She regarded this as an excuse to avoid being attentive to his needs. He had also developed very disfiguring pustules on his face, arms and legs. His father's sister thought people were disgusted by him, and preferred not to spend time with him. She did not, however, agree with me that he should go back to the hospital. He himself was adamant that he wished to stay at home and that he was tired of treatment. His *tete* was of the firm opinion that he needed proper looking after and, for her, this meant close attention to his physical needs but also long periods of time reading the Bible with him, and praying with him. Nicholas was always delighted by her visits.

My experience is that many children chose, at some point, to withdraw from treatment. Priscilla continues to vacillate in her attitudes to her treatment and the form of life that it allows her to keep suffering. The other children I have mentioned who have died have all, at some point, made choices to withdraw from active medical treatment. They have left hospital, discontinued medications and avoided hospital appointments and medical personnel. These discontinuations are often accompanied by a physical withdrawal to the rural home of some part of their family (when such is available, for many urban Zimbabweans either no longer have, or no longer have easy access to, rural homes).

I understand these withdrawals as, in part, decisions to stop struggling, and in part avoidance of the language and implications of failure that medical institutions will place on their decisions to withdraw. Phrases such as 'failure to adhere' carry a freight of the pejorative and, besides, most of the children I know consider the professionals who try to treat their illnesses with the highest regard. They express active and acute concern that their withdrawal will disappoint and distress their medical carers. Amongst children and their immediate carers there is a more subtle exchange of concerns in relation to the decision to withdraw from both life and medical care. A central part of this exchange is that both adults and children operate on a shared, though often unspoken, acceptance of the very hard realities of continuing to struggle for life. Of course, there are exceptions. While Persistence's mother simply cannot bear to see her son cry any more, Priscilla's aunt (as we saw in the chapter on family and kin) is spurred on by the sudden possibility of her death to begin to argue forcefully for the claims of life, not least through a re-animated care and concern.

As we have noted before, many Zimbabwean families have suffered multiple bereavements. The ranks of family members, and wider kin, are often sorely depleted. For example, Persistence's mother knows of only two remaining members on his father's side of the family, and she believes all the rest to have died. And death is not the only cause of depletion within families. The Zimbabwean diaspora is now commonly said to number over three million (out of a total population of approximately 11 million). Family members who seek work outside of the country choose lives of uncertainty and tenuous bonds of communication with those left behind. Here, where loss and absence predominate, it is increasingly difficult to pass on the tasks of caring for survivors. This is a greater concern for adults who are carers.

An epilogue

In a fascinating though difficult paper, *'Cutting the network'*, Marilyn Strathern (1996) draws parallels between various forms of networks, human and not, and the ways in which they might be manipulated socially and analytically. Part of her argument concerns funeral rites in Micronesia and the ways in which death cuts older networks, only to re-animate new ones. I cite her here, though, since she makes a very interesting and I think timely point about pausing:

> In fact, the concept (of network) can conjoin anything, a ubiquity consonant with the ubiquity of culture itself. I see the apprehension of surfeit, then, as a moment of interpretive pause. Interpretation must hold objects of reflection stable long enough to be of use. That holding stable may be imagined as stopping a flow or cutting into an expanse .... Old networks are cut by being gathered up at a point (in the deceased), whose socially hybrid form is dispersed and thereby brings new networks into play. The relationships that once sustained the deceased become recombined in the persons of others. (Strathern 1996: 527)

Some two months ago, Persistence's mother suddenly re-appeared. She had come back to town. It seemed the worst of her grief at the loss of her eldest child had receded. She herself had returned to the clinic and had recently started ARV treatment. She had also decided to have her youngest child tested, even though he had always been healthy. His name is Kudzi, and he is 14. He had tested positive. I was shocked and particularly fearful for how this would affect his mother, whom I had come to see as frail and heavily burdened. She surprised me by her wry, though melancholic, acceptance. 'It is better that we know now,' she said, 'he will get treatment sooner than Persistence did and, anyway, he has always been a stronger boy.' And now would come my chance to display the usefulness that I had longed to find in the wake of Persistence's death, 'and, besides,' she smiled, 'he will have you to help him.' It seems after all that I am to become more than fictive kin. The relationships forged in the course of fieldwork transform themselves into the more enduring bonds of close, kin-like relationships.

Kudzi and his mother had come to invite me to the first year's anniversary of Persistence's death and burial. This is a ritual known as *kurova guva* (to beat the grave) and, in a sense, is the principal funeral rite, taking place a year or more after the death and perceived to be the principal rite by which the spirit is settled and welcomed into the pantheon of family spirits, who from now on will watch over the living members of their family. As we saw earlier in the work of Michael Bourdillon, in times past, it was highly unusual for the rite to be performed for the young and unmarried.[15] Modern times often see the rite performed but now, with a Christian gloss, referred to as 'the placing of the gravestone'. Persistence's mother, however, used the older expression of *kurova guva*, and made a point of telling me that at the time of Persistence's death it had been Kudzi who had first begun to dig the grave, 'crying, and with his bare hands'. She had indeed been to see her local chief precisely in order to obtain permission to carry out the rite for a young, unmarried boy, and had received it.

We travelled to their rural home together in a car overloaded with supplies and neighbours collected along the way. The homestead, when we reached it, was poor and dilapidated. Its only inhabitant was Persistence's elderly grandmother (his mother's mother). Kudzi and his mother were in tears. Neighbours took over the tasks of cooking, and preparing cement for the headstone. Gradually, those

---

[15] For a more detailed account see Bourdillon (1976: 209-210).

attending began to sing Christian hymns. The family are members of the Methodist church and, as Persistence's mother explained to me, 'had always been Christians'. There was no church minister in attendance but prayers were offered by many of those present, along with gifts of money and food to the family (*kuchema*, in tears), and then ritual gifts of water and maize meal (gifts offered to the spirit to please and 'cool' it, so here we have a ritual that mixes the Christian with the traditional in simple ways). The grave was covered with cement, and a simple cross placed at its head. Slowly, the small crowd began to disperse. I asked Mai Persistence how she was feeling. 'Ah,' she replied, 'one day this will all be over.[16] After all, who am I now that my child has gone?'

After Strathern, this is a moment of the surfeit of grief and loss, and an appropriate place for an interpretive pause.

[16] In Shona, *zvichazondipererawo*, which I think has greater impact and starkness than in its English translation.

7
The heart remains
An epilogue

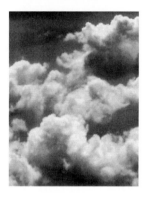

The mbira (a hand-held piano-like instrument, at once percussive and melodic) is quintessentially Shona, even though similar instruments are found throughout Africa. In his classic study of the instrument, and its place in Shona cultures, Paul Berliner (1978) demonstrates how the instrument and its music were not only intrinsic to a local love of music, but were also central to many rituals associated with mourning the dead and honouring their spirits. At the end of his book he gives a number of transcribed lyrics from performances he witnessed (and taped). The vocals accompanying mbira performances are often improvised and so we cannot know how widely known were the examples he gives us. However, he presents the lyrics from a performance by Simon Mashoko in 1971, in the midst of which occurs the following line: '*Kufa ndakuda wasara mwoyo*'. In the book, the well-known Shona language scholars Aaron Hodza and George Fortune give the following translation, 'As far as death is concerned I am ready. What remains is the heart' (Berliner 1978: 256). My own informants gave me another translation, 'I wish to die but my heart remains'. Whatever the best translation, I think the power of the sentiment is clear: death may not seem like a bad thing (particularly when life is filled with pain and suffering), but our emotions feel as though they cannot but remain attached to the people and things of our lives. Our loves may outlive us.

The lyric stayed in my mind for many days, and seems especially pertinent to the work I present here. A study of the lives of children with HIV is a study of suffering and death, grief and hardship. At the same time it is a study of resilience, humour and forbearance under the most extreme of circumstances. In keeping with my declared commitment to an ethic of restraint I do not intend to end with a detailed theoretical analysis of the ethnography I have presented. I will, however, offer some spare reflections that seem to me to be pertinent, and to stand as markers for fuller analysis, either by myself or others, in time to come. Hence the title of 'epilogue' rather than 'conclusion' and, with 'the heart remains', a reminder of emotional surfeit and appropriate interpretive pauses. This work is, perhaps, as much threnody[1] as ethnography.

The ethnography examined the lives of children growing up with HIV in the small, eastern Zimbabwean town of Mutare. The town and some of its more relevant features and experiences were described. Subsequently, children's lives were explored in the contexts of family and kin, clinics and other forms of healing, churches and practices of religious faith and in relation to their deaths and griefs. Each of the domains was explored in relation to what children or their families told me, as well as against templates of other literatures which bear on such experiences. I have tried to foreground children's words or my direct observations of their daily lives. Over the years of the study, it also became possible to make and sustain close relationships with the families and caregivers of the children, many of whom were themselves HIV-positive. These relationships greatly enhanced the usefulness of the group and our understand-

[1] 'Threnody: a single lament emerging from the interactions between multiple wailings and dirges.

ing of the pressures and forms of care available (or not) to the children. Significantly, the life span of the study took place during a major crisis in the Zimbabwean state with the complete collapse of the education system, and the near complete collapse of the health system. Children and their caregivers were struggling with extreme poverty, and widespread social violence. Malnutrition is common and livelihoods extremely precarious. It would seem to be against the spirit of ethnography to attempt a summary of anything we might rightly call 'the major findings' of the study, but such a summary might include some of the following.

Most children were aware of being HIV-positive, and aware of the implications of illness and death, and yet had been brought up in families where the need for absolute secrecy was stressed in relation to their HIV status, primarily in order to protect them from the potentially devastating (and greatly feared) effects of social stigma. Most children and their families were reluctant (but relatively regular) users of antiretrovirals and other life-saving medications, appearing to prefer the possibilities of spiritual healing through (primarily) the explosively growing charismatic churches. There is a worrying disconnect between the teachings of charismatic churches (healing is available to those with sufficient faith) which are the region's fastest growing form of religious belief and practice, and its deadliest infectious disease. Many children view their adherence to medication regimes as a failure of faith. Poverty is a far greater threat to the lives of these children than is HIV. The group is most helpful to children and their families when primary attention is paid to basic needs such as adequate food, shelter, access to clean water, access to education, transport costs and clinic fees.

The concept of 'the orphan' has almost no meaning in southern Africa's histories or cultures. Parenthood has never been locally defined on a strictly biological basis. Children have clear communities of care surrounding them from both paternal and maternal kin, whether their biological parents are alive or dead. There are clear ethical problems in attempting to provide further care to these children in settings and groups with thinly veiled, primary aims of Christian evangelization. This raises questions about the appropriateness of donor reliance on faith-based organizations to provide care. HIV-positive adolescents are sexually active (as are their non-HIV-positive peers). However there is no systematic education on safe sexual practices either in churches or families, and schools remain uncertain sites of valid information.

Mutare is my home and the children and their families remain an important feature of my life. I continue to meet with the group weekly. I have no plans to stop doing so. In the course of a five-year period of fieldwork I have developed close relationships with all of them. In many households I am now treated as a family member, called father or uncle or big brother. I have willingly entered into the transformation of relationships from those of therapeutic clients and ethnographic informants to family membership. The process is mutual. Children and families have offered me the change of role as much as I have accepted it. Extreme discrepancies continue to mark our differences, of course. Class, race, education, age and background (amongst much else) are not so lightly to be done away with. But they have proved less insurmountable than I might have thought five years ago. The transformation of relationships reinforces my determination to uphold an ethical restraint in relation to my knowledge, and my need to honour the dead and dying.

The reflections I offer might be loosely gathered into two groups. The first of these speaks to discourses of HIV, and of the body. The second, to questions of ethnographic and psychotherapeutic method and practice.

Discourses of HIV, and of the body

Immersed in the terrible realities of the HIV epidemic in southern Africa, there are few who now recall that much early AIDS activism was the work of western gay men. Direct action groups like ACT UP and Queer Nation did extraordinary work, at considerable personal cost, to protest the deliberate and homophobic inertia of western states, to promote prevention and to advocate for access to treatments. The blatant profiteering of large transnational pharmaceutical firms was largely exposed through the relentless work of such groups. Many of these men did not live to see the fruits of their labour. One of their most fluent polemicists, Paul Monette wrote, shortly before his death, 'Grief is a sword, or it is nothing' (1994: 115).

The phrase (which I saw printed on T-shirts at Gay Pride parades in the West in the late 1990s) aptly captures some of the profound differences between experiences of the epidemic in the West and in the global south. Even though, with a training in psychotherapy, I disagreed with the statement (grief, it seems to me, is many things, only one of which may be a sword), it very concisely captured the rage that fueled activism and expressed an underlying outrage that citizens were being subject to lethal discrimination. Such entitlement, such a sense of betrayed belonging, would appear not to hold the same traction in most of southern Africa. Outside of South Africa's Treatment Action Campaign[2] (and South Africa, arguably, is a regional exception), southern Africa[3] has not seen the rise of local direct action groups expressing the anger and demands of infected people. The absence of anger can be puzzling. Presenting an earlier version of the chapter on death and dying to a US academic audience, one of the first questions I received was about the absence of rage in dying children. Indeed, I saw none.

So striking a difference suggests causes that are multi-determined. However, one path through the conundrum may lie in thinking about the very different ways in which the body, and corporeality,

[2]   Again, see Iliffe (2006) for a masterly summary of the TAC and its major successes in challenging and overcoming the indifference of the SA government.

[3]   I am only speaking of southern central Africa here.

may be experienced in the West and the global south. Both Neville Hoad (2007) and Beth Povinelli (2006) have begun to develop critical work which suggests that the body and corporeality may be socially constructed and personally experienced as profoundly separate from their (loose) state attachments. The shadow of western, liberal ideologies does not reach very far.[4] Centuries of physical suffering (through, *inter alia*, colonialism, poverty, oppression and violence) construe the experience of the body diversely and render the claims of citizenship remote. Hence the idea of an activism based on the needs of the body loses purchase, and rage (against whom?) becomes pointless, even unthinkable.

The theoretical lens I sketch here therefore also renders much recent anthropology of HIV inexplicable in the southern African context. In particular, the works of João Biehl have presented compelling and influential anthropological accounts of HIV in Brazil. In *Will to Live: AIDS Therapies and the Politics of Survival*, Biehl and Eskerod (2007) provide a compelling social history of AIDS activism in Brazil but a thin account of its failures in relation to the poorest. *Vita: Life in a Zone of Social Abandonment* (2005), his beautiful account of one homeless woman's struggle with apparently terminal illness in a context of unrelenting oppression is, for me, rendered curiously incomprehensible by an end in which poverty and disease, madness and survival, are redeemed through proper medical diagnosis (in this case, genetic neurological degeneration). Much of the confusion can be traced, I suggest, to the influential work of Arthur Kleinman (for example, 1988, 2006), a founder of medical anthropology and cross-cultural psychiatry, which is shot through with covert and confounding tropes of morality, redemption and the powers of western medicine. In Kleinman, western medical science and practice is a remoralizing (unstoppably global) force, which sutures the citizen

---

[4]   See also Sylvia Tamale (2011), an extraordinarily rich collection of essays by African scholars on the deeply under-researched topic of sexuality in Africa.

back into the social fabric, and proper citizenship, through the ethical practice of care, and of care as bearing witness. (The work of Paul Farmer (2003) might also be criticized in similar vein). Kleinman's work is based quite specifically on western medical practice which it valorizes, and under which regime its only limits appear to be those imposed by resource constraints. For anthropological works it is remarkable in its elision of other ideas of the body, or of other regimes of healing which are premised on thoroughly different ideas about the relationships between body, illness and healing. None of this can be taken to be illuminating in the southern African, post-colonial context marked, as it is, by poor governance, poverty and failing states (as well as powerful, socially entrenched and persistent ideas about illness as indicators of disorder between the living and the dead, or between the living and the divine). There can be no medically remoralized citizens in contexts where health services do not function and 'citizens' have lost (or never acquired) the expectation that they might.

I think my study has shown that poor, HIV-infected children in eastern Zimbabwe do not expect, indeed think, to claim rights (including biomedical ones) from the state. They do not claim anything. They do not demand. They seek help primarily through family and kin, and religious structures. The state is remote and largely hostile. Therefore grief, in my work, is not a sword. Neither medical practice (nor infrastructure), nor a sympathetic state, offer people the possibilities of protest. In Mutare, among dreadfully ill children and their families, the form that grief takes lies adjacent to protest – in forms I have yet to give words to – but may be something like despair, or simply struggling on.

Method: ethnographic and psychotherapeutic

The question of whether and how research methods, epistemologies and practices from both psychotherapy and ethnography may be combined in pursuit of enhancing both is an important and urgent one, perhaps more so in times when social suffering greatly bears down on them. I have already, in the study, put forward my view that such an engagement across disciplines suggests a possibility of explicating and easing the lives of children under conditions of severe adversity and allowing possibilities for environments more conducive to growth and development. I should make it clear that I have come to regard most standard forms of the practice of psychotherapy as cultural (western) practices with little to offer in other cultural contexts in their current forms. The divulgence of 'family matters' outside of family domains, the curiosities of the prescribed times and payments of western psychotherapy (themselves highly ritualized), and the emotional remoteness of the therapist are all profoundly alien cultural practices. Furthermore, as I have pointed out, it is entirely unclear in what ways western psychologies can claim to represent, or explain, divergent peoples in thoroughly 'other' cultural contexts.[5] Indeed, when so many of the tenets of psychotherapy are thrown into question, we might ask what remains. A process of companionship? An abandonment of the idea of 'cure'? These are matters deserving extensive, collaborative study in their own right. I regard the work I present here as merely an initial foray into an area that urgently needs more substantial study. I do, however, have some observations to make in this regard.

The work I have described here took a long time to complete. The study ran, intermittently, from 2005 to 2010. The question of timeframes in excess of what are considered usual in anthropology (or psychology) is an important one. The study was concerned with children who are HIV-infected in contexts of potentially devastating social stigma, further confounded by poverty and political oppression. Under such circumstances relationships with informants require sustained investments of time and resources. The value of the information I obtained from children and their families is

[5]   Again, see Burman (2008).

directly related to the depth and resilience of relationships of trust and commitment that were themselves the result of long-term work. It might be the case that both psychotherapy and anthropology have become more attached to shorter-term engagements as a result of consideration of costs and resources, and the pressures to produce 'results' of more immediate value. 'Immediate value' is, of course, a highly problematic category in its own right, as are 'results'.

The information obtained in the course of fieldwork (or of psycho-therapeutic engagement) is frequently extremely painful to hear, to observe and to bear witness to. Therefore we might wonder about how researchers and practitioners might be enabled to bear such listening without rapid, instinctive recourse to 'help' or 'rescue'. For example, many painful incidents I have described in the study would, in western contexts, have elicited (indeed mandated) recourse to legal (specifically child protective) mechanisms. The Zimbabwe-an context only has such resources (and demands) in the abstract. I imagine the same is true in many non-western contexts. How do we bear with uncertainty, danger and risk? How do we bear with the pain of others? (And how do we pass on such abilities and insights to our students who are earlier in their research careers?)

I believe that every chapter of the study suggests lines for further enquiry. I hope that my own long-term engagement with the group of children and their families will allow me to continue to hear their pain, observe their lives, help where I can and commit the knowl-edge gained thereby to further writing, and reflection. For example, the Zimbabwean context continues to deteriorate. In the past two years (as I have been writing) there have been new and deadly outbreaks of measles (like cholera, an entirely preventable disease). There may be others. Another decade may bring material that casts light on children's struggles to live or die, and on the institutions (clinics, churches, families) which support them in doing so. Captur-ing such trajectories will be important for a future, psychologically informed anthropology.

Perhaps most fundamentally, though, I believe my work demonstrates the need for further, considerably more detailed, study of the lexicon of the emotions.[6] Despair, resignation, sorrow and grief, for example, are all words drawn from a western (English) vocabulary and bear the institutional imprints of more than a century of psychoanalytic (indeed psychiatric) work. Any ethnographer (or linguist) will be acutely conscious that words cannot often be directly translated. Yet words are intrinsic to cultural competency and contextual sensitivity. Elsewhere I have drawn attention to ways in which Shona languages render accounts of pain (physical, emotional, spiritual, social) far more complex than is taken into account by contemporary western trauma theory (Parsons 2006). There I examined the many and very subtle ways in which the English word 'pain' was given to me by my informant. The nuances of a variety of Shona words (for example, pain as physical, pain as disruptive of the social, pain of separation) are lost in the direct translation of his account into the solitary English word. Thus attention to linguistic specificity in other cultural contexts enables a serious challenge to hegemonic western emotional lexicons and their real power in forms of western medical (specifically psychiatric) power. We need constantly to be aware that western modes of understanding are not simply alternative views. They drive funding and programming throughout the world, as we have seen, for example, in the case of discourses about 'orphans' or 'trauma'. In this sense they are imbued with substantial power.

Indeed, contemporary critical theory, in particular the recent much vaunted 'turn to affect',[7] is remarkable, for an anthropologist, in its decidedly western philosophical modes and in its lack of atten-

---

[6] And hence my preface to the work, which is a comment from Wittgenstein on the major philosophical problems inherent in giving languaged form to pain and suffering. 'For how can I go so far as to try to use language to get between pain and its expression?' (Wittgenstein 1945: 245)

[7] See Leys (2000, 2007) for a particularly sharp critique of 'affect' in current western critical theory.

tion to linguistic variation (and therefore cultural translatability). I think this is a question of method and also of focus. How are particular emotions named, heard and attached to conditions, persons and events? In what ways would our understanding of affect be altered by attention to the immense variation, and subtle nuances, of the languages of emotion in a plethora of non-western contexts?

After Hurbinek

In Primo Levi's extraordinary, almost unbearable accounts of life in and after the Nazi death camps (1959, 1965, 1988), we find an account of a child called Hurbinek. Frail, wasted and immobile he died of typhoid fever shortly after the liberation of the camps. For Giorgio Agamben (1999) he becomes the ultimate symbol of voiceless witness. A reading of Levi's original account, however, complicates Agamben's elegant polemics, for there we find Hurbinek not to be only (or entirely) an isolated, silent figure but a child deeply embedded in and nurtured by a sociality of other children. Hurbinek is cared for and mourned by other children who have made their own complex barters for survival against appalling odds.[8] I hesitate to invoke the literature of the Holocaust because it is the ultimate

---

[8] '[Henek] was in the bunk next to me, a robust and hearty Hungarian boy of fifteen. Henek spent half his day beside Hurbinek's pallet. He was maternal rather than paternal; had our precarious coexistence lasted more than a month, it is extremely probable that Hurbinek would have learned to speak from Henek … Henek … calm and stubborn, sat beside the little sphinx, immune to the distressing power he emanated; he brought him food to eat, adjusted his blankets, cleaned him with skilful hands, without repugnance; and he spoke to him … in a slow and patient voice.' (Levi 1965: 22); and 'Hurbinek was not the only child. There were others, in relatively good health; they had formed a little "club", very closed and reserved, in which the intrusion of adults was visibly unwelcome. *They were wild and judicious little animals, who conversed in languages I could not understand.* The most authoritative member of the clan was no more than five years old, and his name was Peter Pavel … (He) spoke to nobody and had need of nobody' (Levi 1965: 25. My emphasis).

ethical limit case of our times, and because the mass deaths of contemporary Zimbabwe (not least those of children) have not yet been adequately demonstrated to be due to single causes or perpetrators. Yet I do so because the figure of Hurbinek and his child peers frolic and disturb, agitate and shock where such antics are least expected. And I do so because I wish to shock. It is one of the forms of my memorial for the dead children of Mutare.

My ethnography is about the specificities of children living with HIV in contemporary Zimbabwe. Their lives are crowded with adversity, and shadowed by imminent illness and death. They deserve an adequate account, and a thick description. May this work be a part of that memorial.

Bibliography

Agamben, Giorgio. 2000. *Remnants of Auschwitz: The Witness and the Archive*. New York: Zone Books.

— 1998. *Homo Sacer: Sovereign Power and Bare Life*. Stanford: Stanford University Press.

Alexander, Jocelyn. 2006. *The Unsettled Land: State-making and the Politics of Land in Zimbabwe, 1893-2003*. Oxford: James Currey; Harare: Weaver Press.

Alexander, Jocelyn, JoAnn McGregor and Terence Ranger. 2000. *Violence and Memory: One Hundred Years in the 'Dark Forests' of Matabeleland*. Oxford: James Currey; Harare: Weaver Press.

Amnesty International. 2011. *220,000 Children: Creating a Lost Generation in Zimbabwe*. http://blog.amnestyusa.org/escr/22000-children-creating-a-lost-generation-in-zimbabwe. Accessed 13 October 2011.

Anderson, Benedict. 1983. *Imagined Communities: Reflections on the Origin and Spread of Nationalism*. London and New York: Verso.

Antze. Paul, and Michael Lambek (eds). 1996. *Tense Past: Cultural Essays in Trauma and Memory*. New York: Routledge.

Aries, Philippe. 1962. *Centuries of Childhood: A Social History of Family Life*. New York: Vintage Books.

Aschwanden, Herbert. 1989. *Karanga Mythology: An Analysis of the Consciousness of the Karanga in Zimbabwe*. Gweru: Mambo Press.

— 1987. *Symbols of Death: An Analysis of the Consciousness of the Karanga*. Gweru: Mambo Press.

Ashforth, Adam. 2005. *Madumo: A Man Bewitched*. Chicago: University of Chicago Press.

— 2005. *Witchcraft, Violence, and Democracy in South Africa*. Chicago: University of Chicago Press.

Barber, Karin. 2007. *The Anthropology of Texts, Persons and Publics: Oral and Written Culture in Africa and Beyond*. New York: Cambridge University Press.

Bateson, Gregory. 1972. *Steps to an Ecology of Mind: Collected Essays in Anthropology, Psychiatry, Evolution, and Epistemology*. San Francisco: Chandler Publishing Company.

— 1965 (1932). *Naven: A Survey of the Problems suggested by a Composite Picture of the Culture of a New Guinea Tribe drawn from Three Points of View*. Stanford: Stanford University Press.

Beach, David. 1994. *The Shona and their Neighbours*. Oxford: Oxford University Press.

— 1994a. 'A Zimbabwean Past: Shona Dynastic Histories and Oral Traditions'. *Zambeziana*. Vol. 21. Gweru: Mambo Press.

— 1980. *The Shona and Zimbabwe, 900-1850: An Outline of Shona History*. New York: Holmes and Meier.

Berliner, Paul. 1978. *The Soul of Mbira: Music and traditions of the Shona people of Zimbabwe*. Berkeley: University of California Press.

Biehl, João Guilherme. 2005. *Vita: Life in a Zone of Social Abandonment*. Berkeley: University of California Press.

Biehl, João Guilherme, and Torben Eskerod. 2007. *Will to Live: AIDS Therapies and the Politics of Survival*. Princeton: Princeton University Press.

Biehl, João Guilherme, Byron Good, and Arthur Kleinman. 2007. *Subjectivity: Ethnographic Investigations*. Berkeley: University of California Press.

Blanchot, Maurice. 1995. *The Writing of the Disaster*. (Trans. A. Smock.)

Lincoln: University of Nebraska Press.

Bluebond-Langner, Myra. 1978. *The Private Worlds of Dying Children*. Princeton: Princeton University Press.

Borneman, John. 2001. 'Caring and Being Cared for: Displacing Marriage, Kinship, Gender and Sexuality'. In James Faubion (ed.), *The Ethics of Kinship*. New Jersey: Rowland and Littlefield.

Bornstein, Erica. 2006. Rituals without Final Acts: Prayer and Success in World Vision Zimbabwe's Humanitarian Work. In Matthew Engelke and Matt Tomlinson (eds), *The Limits of Meaning: Case Studies in the Anthropology of Christianity*. New York: Berghahn Books.

— 2005. *The Spirit of Development: Protestant NGOs, Morality, and Economics in Zimbabwe*. Stanford: Stanford University Press.

Bourdillon, Michael. 2010. Personal communication.

— 1994. 'Street Children in Harare'. *Africa* 64, 4: 516-32.

— 1991. *Poor, Harassed but Very Much Alive: An Account of Street People and their Organization*. Gweru: Mambo Press.

Bourdillon, Michael. 1976. *The Shona Peoples: An Ethnography of the Contemporary Shona, with Special Reference to their Religion*. Gweru: Mambo Press.

Bucher, Hubert. 1980. *Spirits and power: An Analysis of Shona Cosmology*. New York: Oxford University Press.

Bullock, Charles. 1928. *The Mashona (The Indigenous Natives of S. Rhodesia)*. Cape Town and Johannesburg: Juta.

Burman, Erica. 2008. *Deconstructing Developmental Psychology*. London and New York: Routledge.

Cannell, Fenella (ed.). 2006. *The Anthropology of Christianity*. Durham: Duke University Press.

Carsten, Janet. 2004. *After Kinship*. Cambridge and New York: Cambridge University Press.

— 1997. *The Heat of the Hearth: The Process of Kinship in a Malay Fishing Community*. Oxford: Clarendon Press.

Castaneda, Claudia. 2002. *Figurations: Child, Bodies, Worlds*. Durham: Duke University Press.

Cohen, David William, and E. S. Atieno Odhiambo. 1992. *Burying SM:*

The Politics of Knowledge and the Sociology of Power in Africa. London: James Currey.

Collier, Jane Fishburne, Sylvia Junko Yanagisako. 1987. *Gender and Kinship: Essays Toward a Unified Analysis*. Stanford: Stanford University Press.

Colson, Elizabeth. 2000. 'The Father as Witch'. *Africa:* 70, 3: 333-58.

Comaroff, Jean, and John L. Comaroff. 1991. *Of Revelation and Revolution*. Chicago: University of Chicago Press.

Comaroff, John L., and Jean Comaroff. 1992. *Ethnography and the Historical Imagination*. Boulder: Westview Press.

Crapanzano, Vincent. 1985. *Tuhami: Portrait of a Moroccan*. Chicago: University of Chicago Press.

Csordas, Thomas J. 1994. *Embodiment and Experience: The Existential Ground of Culture and Self*. Cambridge and New York: Cambridge University Press.

Dalai Lama, The. 1999. *Ancient Wisdom, Modern World: Ethics for a New Millennium*. London: Little, Brown.

Daneel, Marthinus L. 1971. *Old and New in Southern Shona Independent Churches*. The Hague: Mouton.

Das, Veena. 2007. *Life and Words: Violence and the Descent into the Ordinary*. Berkeley: University of California Press.

— 1996. 'Violence and the Work of Time'. In Anthony Cohen (ed.), *Signifying Identities: Anthropological Perspectives on Boundaries and Contested Values*. London: Routledge.

— 1990. 'Our Work to Cry, Your Work to Listen'. In Veena Das (ed.), *Mirrors of Violence: Communities, Riots and Survivors in South Asia*. Delhi: Oxford University Press.

Das, Veena, and Pamela Reynolds. 2003. 'The Child on the Wing: Children Negotiating the Everyday in the Geography of Violence'. Unpublished paper, Department of Anthropology, Johns Hopkins University.

De Baets, Anniek, Sibongile Sifovo, Ross Parsons, and Isidore Pazvakavambwa. 2008. 'HIV Disclosure and Discussions about Grief with Shona Children: A Comparison between Health Care Workers and

Community Members in Eastern Zimbabwe'. *Social Science and Medicine* 66: 479-91.

De Boeck, Filip. 1998. 'Domesticating Diamonds and Dollars: Identity, Expenditure and Sharing in Southwestern Zaire (1984-1997)'. *Development and Change* 29, 4: 777-810.

De Boeck, Filip, and Marie-Francoise Plissart. 2004. *Kinshasa: Tales of the Invisible City.* Ghent: Ludion.

Deleuze, Gilles and Felix Guattari. 1987 (1980). *A Thousand Plateaus: Capitalism and Schizophrenia.* (Trans. Brian Massumi.) Minneapolis: University of Minnesota University Press.

Desjarlais, Robert R. 2003. *Sensory Biographies: Lives and Deaths among Nepal's Yolmo Buddhists.* Berkeley: University of California Press.

— 1993. *Body and Emotion: The Aesthetics of Illness and Healing in the Nepal Himalayas.* Philadelphia: University of Pennsylvania Press.

Devisch, Renaat, and Claude Brodeur. 1999. *The Law of the Lifegivers: The Domestication of Desire.* Amsterdam: Harwood Academic.

Douglas, Mary. 1966. *Purity and Danger: An Analysis of Concepts of Pollution and Taboo.* London: Penguin.

Engelke, Matthew. 2002. 'The Problem of Belief: Evans-Pritchard and Victor Turner on "the Inner Life".' *Anthropology Today* 18, 6: 3-8.

Engelke, Matthew, and Matt Tomlinson (eds). 2006. *The Limits of Meaning: Case Studies in the Anthropology of Christianity.* New York: Berghahn Books.

Evans-Pritchard, Edward. 1962. *Essays in Social Anthropology.* London: Faber and Faber.

— 1962. 'Religion and the Anthropologists: The Aquinas Lecture 1959'. In Evans-Pritchard, *Essays in Social Anthropology.* London: Faber and Faber.

Fanon, Franz. 1961 (1965). *The Wretched of the Earth.* London: Penguin.

Farmer, Paul. 2003. *Pathologies of Power: Health, Human Rights, and the New War on the Poor.* Berkeley: University of California Press.

Feierman, Steven, and John M. Janzen. 1992. *The Social Basis of Health and Healing in Africa.* Berkeley: University of California Press.

Ferenczi, Sándor. 1955. *Final Contributions to the Problems and Methods of*

Psycho-analysis. New York: Basic Books.

Ferguson, James. 2006. *Global Shadows: Africa in the Neoliberal World Order.* Durham: Duke University Press.

— 1999. *Expectations of Modernity: Myths and Meanings of Urban Life on the Zambian Copperbelt.* Berkeley: University of California Press.

Fernandez, James W. 1982. *Bwiti: An Ethnography of the Religious Imagination in Africa.* Princeton: Princeton University Press.

Foster, Geoff, Carol Levine, and John Williamson. 2005. *A Generation at Risk: The Global Impact of HIVAIDS on Orphans and Vulnerable Children.* Cambridge and New York: Cambridge University Press.

Freud, Sigmund. 1915. 'Thoughts for the Times on War and Death'. In James Strachey (ed. and trans.), *The Standard Edition of the Complete Psychological Works of Sigmund Freud.* London: Hogarth Press.

— 2003 [1917]. *Beyond the Pleasure Principle and Other Writings.* London and New York: Penguin.

— 2003 [1921]. *On Mourning and Melancholia.* London: Penguin.

Geertz, Clifford. 2000. *Available light: Anthropological Reflections on Philosophical Topics.* Princeton: Princeton University Press.

— 1983. *Local Knowledge: Further Essays in Interpretive Anthropology.* New York: Basic Books.

— 1973. *The Interpretation of Cultures: Selected Essays.* New York: Basic Books.

Gelfand, Michael. 1979. *Growing up in Shona Society: From Birth to Marriage.* Gwelo: Mambo Press.

— 1967. *The African Witch.* Edinburgh: E. and S. Livingstone.

Geschiere, Peter, and Janet Roitman. 1997. *The Modernity of Witchcraft: Politics and the Occult in Postcolonial Africa.* Charlottesville: University of Virginia Press.

Gluckman, Max. 1955. *The Judicial Process among the Barotse of Northern Rhodesia.* Manchester: Manchester University Press, on behalf of the Rhodes-Livingstone Institute, Northern Rhodesia.

Haase, Ulrich, and William Large. 2001. *Maurice Blanchot.* London: Routledge.

Hammar, Amanda. 2010. 'Ambivalent Mobilities: Zimbabwean Commercial Farmers in Mozambique'. *Journal of Southern African Studies* 36, 2: 395-416.

Hammar, Amanda, JoAnn McGregor and Loren Landau. 2010. 'Displacing Zimbabwe: Crisis and Construction in Southern Africa'. *Journal of Southern African Studies* 36, 2: 263-84.

Hammar, Amanda, Brian Raftopoulos, and Stig Jensen (eds). 2003. *Zimbabwe's Unfinished Business: Rethinking Land, State and Nation in the Context of Crisis*. Harare: Weaver Press.

Hamutyinei, M and A Plangger. 1974. *Tsumo-Shumo: Shona Proverbial Lore and Wisdom*. Gweru: Mambo Press.

Harold-Barry, David (ed.). 2004. *Zimbabwe: The Past is the Future*. Harare: Weaver Press.

Hart, Jason. 2006. 'Saving Children: What Role for Anthropology?' *Anthropology Today* 22, 1: 5-8.

Heald, Suzette. 1988. *Controlling Anger: The Sociology of Gisu Violence*. Manchester: Manchester University Press.

Heald, Suzette, and Ariane Deluz. 1994. *Anthropology and Psychoanalysis: An Encounter through Culture*. London and New York: Routledge.

Hejoaka, Fabienne. 2009. 'Care and Secrecy: Being a Mother of Children Living with HIV in Burkina Faso'. *Social Science and Medicine* 41: 1-8.

Henderson, Patricia. 2004. 'The Vertiginous Body and Social Metamorphosis in a Context of HIV/AIDS'. *Anthropology Southern Africa* 27, 1-2: 43-53.

Hoad, Neville. 2007. *African Intimacies: Race, Homosexuality, and Globalization*. Minneapolis: University of Minnesota Press.

Hodza, Aaron C., and George Fortune. 1979. *Shona Praise Poetry*. Oxford: Clarendon Press.

Holleman Johan Frederik. 1969. *Chief, Council and Commissioner: Some Problems of Government in Rhodesia*. London, Oxford University Press.

— 1952. *Shona Customary Law, with Reference to Kinship, Marriage, the Family and the Estate*. Cape Town, London and New York: Oxford University Press.

Honwana, Alcinda Manuel. 2006. *Child Soldiers in Africa*. Philadelphia:

University of Pennsylvania Press.

Honwana, Alcinda, and Filip de Boeck. 2005. *Makers and Breakers: Children and Youth in Postcolonial Africa*. Oxford: James Currey.

Hughes, David McDermott. 1999. 'Refugees and Squatters: Immigration and the Politics of Territory on the Zimbabwe-Mozambique Border'. *Journal of Southern African Studies* 25, 4: 533-52.

Iliffe, John. 2006. *The African AIDS Epidemic: A History*. Athens: Ohio University Press; Oxford: James Currey.

Jones, Jeremy. 2010. '"Nothing is Straight in Zimbabwe": The Rise of the Kukiya-kiya Economy 2000-2008'. *Journal of Southern African Studies* 36, 2: 285-300.

Kardiner, Abram, and Ralph Linton. 1939. *The Individual and His Society; The Psychodynamics of Primitive Social Organization*. New York: Columbia University Press.

Keane, Webb. 2007. *Christian Moderns: Freedom and Fetish in the Mission Encounter*. Berkeley: University of California Press.

Kinsey, Bill. 2010. 'Who Went Where ... and Why: Patterns and Consequences of Displacement in Rural Zimbabwe after February 2000'. *Journal of Southern African Studies* 36, 2: 339-60.

— 2006. 'Epilogue: Anxious Transcendence'. In Fenella Cannell (ed.), *The Anthropology of Christianity*. Durham: Duke University Press.

Kleber, Rolf, Charles Figley and Berthold Gersons (eds). 1995. *Beyond Trauma: Cultural and Societal Dynamics*. New York: Plenum Press.

Kleinman, Arthur. 2006. *What Really Matters: Living a Moral Life amidst Uncertainty and Danger*. Oxford and New York: Oxford University Press.

— 1988. *The Illness Narratives: Suffering, Healing, and the Human Condition*. New York: Basic Books.

Kriger, Norma J. 2003. *Guerrilla Veterans in Post-War Zimbabwe: Symbolic and Violent Politics, 1980-1987*. New York: Cambridge University Press.

Kübler-Ross, Elisabeth. 1969. *On Death and Dying*. New York: Macmillan.

Lan, David. 1985. *Guns and Rain: Guerrillas and Spirit Mediums in Zimbabwe*. London: James Currey.

Leach, Edmund. 1961. *Rethinking Anthropology*. London: Athlone Press.

Leibnitz, Gottfried. 1710 (1985). *Théodicée*. (Trans. Austin Farrer and E.M. Huggard.) Wiener III.11 (part). A translation is available at Project Gutenberg.

Levi, Primo. 1988. *The Drowned and the Saved*. (Trans. Raymond Rosenthal.) New York: Orion Press.

— 1965. *The Truce: A Survivor's Journey Home from Auschwitz*. (Trans. Stuart Woolf.) London: Bodley Head.

— 1959. *If This is a Man*. (Trans. Stuart Woolf.) New York: Orion Press.

Leys, Ruth. 2007. *From Guilt to Shame: Auschwitz and After*. Princeton: Princeton University Press.

— 2000. *Trauma: A Genealogy*. Chicago: University of Chicago Press.

Lifton, Robert Jay. 1991. Death in Life: Survivors of H*iroshima*. Chapel Hill: University of North Carolina Press.

Lindemann, Erich. 1979. *Beyond Grief: Studies in Crisis Intervention*. New York: Aronson.

Linden, Ian. 1979. *Church and State in Rhodesia, 1959-1979*. Kaiser, Grunewald.

Lopman, Ben, James Lewis, Constance Nyamukapa, Phyllis Mushati, Steven Chandiwana, and Simon Gregson. 2007. 'HIV Incidence and Poverty in Manicaland, Zimbabwe: Is HIV Becoming a Disease of the Poor?' *AIDS* 21, 7: 557-66.

Lutz, Catherine. 1988. *Unnatural emotions: Everyday Sentiments on a Micronesian Atoll and their Challenge to Western Theory*. Chicago: University of Chicago Press.

Lutz, Catherine, and Geoffrey White. 1986. 'The Anthropology of Emotions'. *Annual Review of Anthropology* 15: 405-36.

Magaramombe, Godfrey. 2010. 'Displaced in Place: Agrarian Displacements, Replacements and Resettlement among Farm Workers in Mazowe District'. *Journal of Southern African Studies* 36, 2: 361-376.

Malinowski, Bronislaw. 1966. *The Father in Primitive Psychology*. New York: Norton.

Marcus, George. 2010. 'Experts, Reporters, Witnesses: The Making of Anthropologists in States of Emergency'. In Didier Fassin and Mariella Pandolfi (eds), *Contemporary States of Emergency: The Politics of*

Military and Humanitarian Interventions. New York: Zone Books.

Mauss, Marcel. 1967 (1925). *The Gift: Forms and Functions of Exchange in Archaic Societies*. New York: Norton.

Mawowa, Showers, and Alois Matongo. 2010. 'Inside Zimbabwe's Roadside Currency Trade: the "World Bank" of Bulawayo'. *Journal of Southern African Studies* 36, 2: 319-38.

Maxwell, David. 2006. *African Gifts of the Spirit: Pentecostalism and the Rise of a Zimbabwean Transnational Religious Movement*. Oxford: James Currey; Harare: Weaver Press.

— 2000. 'Catch the Cockerel before Dawn: Pentecostalism and Politics in Postcolonial Zimbabwe'. *Africa* 70, 2: 249-77.

Mazarire, Gerald. 2009. Reflections on Pre-Colonial Zimbabwe, c.850-1880s. In Brian Raftopoulos and Alois Mlambo (eds), *Becoming Zimbabwe: A History from the Pre-colonial Period to 2008*. Harare: Weaver Press, Harare.

Mbembe, Achille. 2002. 'African Modes of Self Writing'. *Public Culture* 14, 1: 239-73.

— 2001. *On the Postcolony*. Berkeley: University of California Press.

Mbembe, Achille, and Janet Roitman. 1995. 'Figures of the Subject in Times of Crisis'. *Public Culture* 7, 2: 323-52.

Mead, Margaret. 1928. *Coming of Age in Samoa; A Psychological Study of Primitive Youth for Western Civilization*. New York: W. Morrow and Company.

Meintjies, Helen, and Sonja Giese. 2006. 'Spinning the Epidemic: The Making of Mythologies of Orphanhood in the Context of AIDS. *Childhood* 13,1: 407-30.

Menzies-Lyth, Isabella. 1988. *Containing Anxiety in Institutions*. London: Free Association Books.

Meyer, Birgit. 1999. *Translating the Devil: Religion and Modernity among the Ewe in Ghana*. Edinburgh: Edinburgh University Press.

Mlambo, Alois. 2009. 'From the Second World War to UDI, 1940-1965'. In Brian Raftopoulos and Alois Mlambo (eds), *Becoming Zimbabwe: A History from the Pre-colonial Period to 2008*. Harare: Weaver Press.

Monette, Paul. 1994. *Last Watch of the Night: Essays Too Personal and Oth-*

erwise. New York: Harcourt, Brace.

Moore, Donald S. 2005. *Suffering for Territory: Race, Place, and Power in Zimbabwe*. Durham: Duke University Press; Harare: Weaver Press.

Moore, Henrietta. 2007. *The Subject of Anthropology: Gender, Symbolism and Psychoanalysis*. Cambridge: Polity Press.

Morris, Rosalind C. 1995. 'All Made Up: Performance Theory and the New Anthropology of Sex and Gender'. *Annual Review of Anthropology* 24: 567-92.

Mtisi, Joseph, Munyaradzi Nyakudya, and Theresa Barnes. 2009. 'Social and Economic Developments during the UDI Period'. In Brian Raftopoulos and Alois Mlambo (eds), *Becoming Zimbabwe: A History from the Pre-colonial Period to 2008*. Harare: Weaver Press.

— 2009. 'War in Rhodesia, 1965-1980'. In Brian Raftopoulos and Alois Mlambo (eds), *Becoming Zimbabwe: A History from the Pre-colonial Period to 2008*. Harare: Weaver Press.

Musoni, Francis. 2010. Operation Murambatsvina and the Politics of Street Vendors in Zimbabwe. *Journal of Southern African Studies* 36, 2: 301-38.

Mutongi, Kenda. 2007. *Worries of the Heart: Widows, Family, and Community in Kenya*. Chicago: University of Chicago Press.

Muzondidya, James. 2009. 'From Buoyancy to Crisis, 1980-1997'. In Brian Raftopoulos and Alois Mlambo (eds), *Becoming Zimbabwe: A History from the Pre-colonial Period to 2008*. Harare: Weaver Press.

Ndhlovu-Gatsheni, Sabelo. 2009. 'Mapping Cultural and Colonial Encounters, 1880s-1930s'. In Brian Raftopoulos and Alois Mlambo (eds), *Becoming Zimbabwe: A History from the Pre-colonial Period to 2008*. Harare: Weaver Press.

Nieuwenhuys, Olga. 1996. 'The Paradox of Child Labor and Anthropology'. *Annual Review of Anthropology* 25: 237-51.

Orner, Peter, and Annie Holmes. 2010. *Hope Deferred: Narratives of Zimbabwean Lives*. San Francisco: McSweeney Books.

Palgi, Phyllis, and Henry Abramovitch. 1984. 'Death: A Cross-Cultural Perspective'. *Annual Review of Anthropology* 13: 385-417.

Parker, Richard. 2001. 'Sexuality, Culture and Power in HIV/AIDS

Research'. *Annual Review of Anthropology* 30: 163-79.

Parsons, Ross. 2010. '"Eating in Mouthfuls while Facing the Door": Some Notes on Childhoods and their Displacements in Eastern Zimbabwe'. *Journal of Southern African Studies* 36, 2: 449-63.

— 2006. 'Troubling Language: Rereading a Narrative of Trauma from Political Violence in Contemporary Zimbabwe'. *International Journal of Critical Psychology* 17: 29-46.

— 2005. Grief-stricken: Zimbabwean Children in Everyday Extremity and the Ethics of Research. *Anthropology Southern Africa* 28, 3/4: 73-7.

Parsons, Ross, Cally Farrell, and Sandy Frangoulis. 2003. 'At the Boiling Point of the Pain: Assessing the Need for a Psychotherapy Service for Victims of Torture and Organized Violence through Attention to the Narratives of Survivors'. Harare: Amani Trust.

Peletz, Michael G. 1995. 'Kinship Studies in Late Twentieth-Century Anthropology'. *Annual Review of Anthropology* 24: 343-72.

Pels, Peter. 1997. 'The Anthropology of Colonialism: Culture, History, and the Emergence of Western Governmentality'. *Annual Review of Anthropology* 26: 163-83.

Pfeiffer, James. 2005. 'Commodity Fetichismo, The Holy Spirit, and the Turn to Pentecostal and African Independent Churches in Central Mozambique'. *Culture, Medicine and Psychiatry* 31: 321-43.

Phillips, Adam. 2000. *Darwin's Worms*. New York: Basic Books.

— 1993. *On Kissing, Tickling, and Being Bored: Psychoanalytic Essays on the Unexamined Life*. Cambridge: Harvard University Press.

Physicians for Human Rights. 2009. *Health in Ruins: A Man-Made Disaster in Zimbabwe*. Cambridge, MA: Physicians for Human Rights.

Povinelli, Beth. 2006. *The Empire of Love: Toward a Theory of Intimacy, Genealogy and Carnality*. Durham: Duke University Press.

Radcliffe-Brown, Alfred R., and Daryll Forde (eds) 1950. *African Systems of Kinship and Marriage*. London: Oxford University Press.

Raftopoulos, Brian. 2009. 'The Crisis in Zimbabwe, 1998-2008'. In Brian Raftopoulos and Alois Mlambo (eds), *Becoming Zimbabwe: A History from the Pre-colonial Period to 2008*. Harare: Weaver Press.

Raftopoulos, Brian, and Alois Mlambo (eds). 2009. *Becoming Zimbabwe:*

A History from the Pre-colonial Period to 2008. Harare: Weaver Press.

Raftopoulos, Brian, and Tyrone Savage (eds). 2005. *Zimbabwe: Injustice and Political Reconciliation*. Harare: Weaver Press.

Ranger, Terence. 1999. *Voices from the Rocks: Nature, Culture and History in the Matopos Hills of Zimbabwe*. Oxford: James Currey; Harare: Baobab Books.

— 1985. *Peasant Consciousness and Guerrilla War in Zimbabwe: A Comparative Study*. London: James Currey.

Ranger, Terence, and Paul Slack. 1992. *Epidemics and Ideas: Essays on the Historical Perception of Pestilence*. Cambridge: Cambridge University Press.

Reeler, Tony. 2004. 'Sticks and Stones, Skeletons and Ghosts'. In David Harold-Barry (ed.) *Zimbabwe: The Past is the Future*. Harare: Weaver Press.

Reynolds, Pamela. 2000. 'The Ground of all Making: State Violence, the Family and Political Activists'. In Veena Das, Arthur Kleinman, Mamphela Ramphele and Pamela Reynolds (eds), *Violence and Subjectivity*. Berkeley: University of California Press.

— 1996. *Traditional Healers and Childhood in Zimbabwe*. Athens: Ohio University Press.

— 1995. '"Not Known Because not Looked for": Ethnographers Listening to the Young in Southern Africa'. *Ethnos* 60, 3-4: 193-221.

— 1991. *Dance, Civet Cat: Child Labour in the Zambezi Valley*. London: Zed Books.

Richards, Audrey I. 1956. *Chisungu: A Girl's' Initiation Ceremony Among the Bemba of Northern Rhodesia*. New York: Grove Press.

— 1939. *Land, Labour and Diet in Northern Rhodesian: An Economic Study of the Bemba Tribe*. Oxford: Oxford University Press.

Rivers, William H.R. 1926. *Psychology and Ethnology*. New York: Harcourt, Brace.

Robbins, Joel. 2004. *Becoming Sinners: Christianity and Moral Torment in a Papua New Guinea Society*. Berkeley: University of California Press.

— 2004a. 'The Globalization of Pentecostal and Charismatic Christianity'. *Annual Review of Anthropology* 33: 117-43.

Ross, Fiona C. 2003. *Bearing Witness: Women and the Truth and Reconciliation Commission in South Africa*. London: Pluto Press.

Rurevo, Rumbidzai and Michael Bourdillon. 2003. *Girls on the Street*. Harare: Weaver Press.

Russ, Ann J. 2005. Love's Labour Paid for: Gift and Commodity at the Threshold of Death'. *Cultural Anthropology* 20, 1: 128-55.

Ryle, Gilbert. 1971. 'Thinking and reflecting'. *Collected Papers*. New York: Barnes and Noble.

Sahlins, Marshall. 1996. 'The Sadness of Sweetness: The Native Anthropology of Western Cosmology. *Current Anthropology* 37, 3: 395.

— 1993. 'Goodbye to *Tristes Tropiques*: Ethnography in the Context of Modern World History'. *The Journal of Modern History* 65, 1: 1-25.

Sapir, Edward. 1949. *Selected Writings of Edward Sapir in Language, Culture and Personality*. Berkeley: University of California Press.

Scheper-Hughes, Nancy. 1992. *Death Without Weeping: The Violence of Everyday Life in Brazil*. Berkeley: University of California Press.

Scheper-Hughes, Nancy, and Carolyn Sargent. 1998. *Small Wars: The Cultural Politics of Childhood*. Berkeley: University of California Press.

Schneider, David Murray. 1968. *American Kinship: A Cultural Account*. Englewood Cliffs, NJ: Prentice-Hall.

Schoepf, Brooke. 2001. 'International AIDS Research in Anthropology: Taking a Critical Perspective on the Crisis'. *Annual Review of Anthropology* 30, 335-61.

Schumaker, Lyn. 2001. *Africanizing Anthropology: Fieldwork, Networks, and the Making of Cultural Knowledge in Central Africa*. Durham: Duke University Press.

Sedgwick, Eve Kosofsky. 2003. *Touching Feeling: Affect, Pedagogy, Performativity*. Durham: Duke University Press.

Solidarity Peace Trust. 2000/2010. Various Reports. www.solidaritypeacetrust.org. Accessed 6 October 2011.

Strathern, Marilyn. 1996. 'Cutting the Network'. *Journal of the Royal Anthropological Institute* 2, 3: 517-35.

Steinberg, Jonny. 2008. *Three Letter Plague*. Cape Town: Jonathan Ball.

Tamale, Sylvia (ed.). 2011. *African Sexualities: A Reader*. Nairobi: Pambazuka Press.

Targoff, Ramie. 2001. *Common Prayer: The Language of Public Devotion in Early Modern England*. Chicago: University of Chicago Press.

Thoreau, Henry David. 1995 (1862). *Walden*. Boston: Houghton Mifflin.

Trawick, Margaret. 1990. *Notes on Love in a Tamil family*. Berkeley: University of California Press.

Turner, Victor Witter. 1981. *The Drums of Affliction: A Study of Religious Processes among the Ndembu of Zambia*. Ithaca, NY: Cornell University Press.

— 1967. *The Forest of Symbols; Aspects of Ndembu Ritual*. Ithaca, NY: Cornell University Press.

van Onselen, Charles. 1996. *The Seed is Mine: The Life of Kas Maine, a South African Sharecropper, 1894-1985*. Oxford: James Currey.

Weber, Max. 1905 (2002). *The Protestant Ethic and the Spirit of Capitalism*. (Trans. Stephen Kalberg.) Los Angeles: Roxbury.

Werbner, Richard. 1997. 'The Suffering Body: Passion and Ritual Allegory in Christian Encounters'. *Journal of Southern African Studies* 23, 2 (Special Issue for Terry Ranger): 311-24.

— 1991. *Tears of the Dead: The Social Biography of an African Family*. Edinburgh: Edinburgh University Press.

— 1984. The Manchester School in South-Central Africa. *Annual Review of Anthropology* 13: 157-85.

— 1977. *Regional cults*. A.S.A. monograph, 16. London and New York: Academic Press.

Werbner, Richard, and Terence Ranger. 1996. *Postcolonial Identities in Africa*. London: Zed Books.

Winnicott, D. W. 1958. *Collected Papers: Through Paediatrics to Psycho-Analysis*. New York: Basic Books.

Wittgenstein, Ludwig. 1945. *Philosophical Investigations*. (Trans. G.E.M Anscombe, 1958.) Third Edition. New Jersey: Prentice Hall.

Worby, Eric. 2010. 'Address Unknown: The Temporality of Displacement and the Ethics of Disconnection among Zimbabwean Migrants in Johannesburg'. *Journal of Southern African Studies* 36, 2: 417-32.

World Bank, The. 2000-2010. Annual Reports: Zimbabwe.

Yourcenar, Marguerite. 1984 (1929). *Alexis.* (Trans. Walter Kaiser.) New York: Farrar, Strauss and Giroux.

Zimbabwe, Ministry of Health and Child Welfare and UNICEF. 2009. 'Preliminary Multiple Indicator Monitoring Survey Report'. Harare: MoHCW/UNICEF.